Aquatic Therapy

INTERVENTIONS AND APPLICATIONS

Luis G. Vargas, Ph.D., P.T.

Idyll Arbor, Inc.

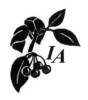

Idyll Arbor, Inc.

PO Box 720, Ravensdale, WA 98051 (425) 432-3231

Idyll Arbor, Inc. Editor: joan burlingame
Idyll Arbor, Inc. Staff Assistant: Bonnie Henry

To the best of our knowledge, the information and recommendations of this book reflect currently accepted practice. Nevertheless, they cannot be considered absolute and universal. Guidelines suggested by federal law are subject to change as the laws and interpretations do. Recommendations for a particular patient must be considered in light of the patient's needs and condition. The editors, author, and publisher disclaim responsibly for any adverse effects resulting directly or indirectly from the suggested therapy practices, from any undetected errors, or from the reader's misunderstanding of the text.

Library of Congress Cataloging-in-Publication Data

Vargas, Luis G., 1953-
  Aquatic therapy : interventions and applications / Luis G. Vargas.
        p. ; cm.
Includes bibliographical references and index.
  ISBN 1-882883-54-3 (hardcover : alk. paper)
  1. Aquatic exercises--Therapeutic use.
  [DNLM: 1. Hydrotherapy--methods. WB 520 V298a 2004] I. Title.
  RM813.V37 2004
  615.8'53--dc22

                                                              2003024177

ISBN 1-882883-54-3

Table of Contents

Table of Figures

ix

x

INTRODUCTION

Aquatic therapy is the process of working with patients to actively or passively rehabilitate musculoskeletal, neurological, and/or cardiopulmonary conditions using water and a pool as the primary therapeutic medium. In this process the therapist observes therapeutic water temperature ranges and applies techniques and interventions to restore function and decrease limitations and pain.

Aquatic therapy has two primary objectives: to facilitate and to inhibit. The use of therapeutic exercise programs and protocols for specific clinical problems and the application of specialized manual techniques or maneuvers help achieve treatment goals. The properties and biophysical laws of water, the relative density of the patient and the medium, and the principles of hydrodynamics are contributing factors that facilitate motor activity in order to improve gait, balance, strength, range of motion, and posture, and inhibit pain, tone, and spasmodic activity. The attainment of these functional and symptomatic objectives depends on the patient's diagnosis, identified clinical problems, and choice of treatment modalities.

There is a difference between aquatic therapy and hydrotherapy. Although both use water as the therapeutic medium and both establish therapeutic temperature ranges, aquatic therapy is a specialized area of clinical concentration that requires advanced knowledge and skill in the application of problem-specific interventions, techniques, and protocols. As a modality, hydrotherapy is a more technical approach to treatment, which has historically focused on the use of mechanical turbines and tanks to produce a hydromassage in the tissues and secondary effects on pain, muscle spasms, and debridement of necrotic tissue.

Some of the functional goals and objectives where aquatic therapy interventions have proven successful include but are not limited to:

1. improvement in motor control
2. improvement in cardiovascular and pulmonary endurance
3. increase in joint range of motion
4. increase in joint flexibility and mobility
5. improvement in postural awareness and alignment
6. decrease in pain
7. resolution of muscle spasms
8. improvement in muscle strength
9. attainment of relaxation
10. improvement in tidal volume and vital capacity
11. reduction in muscle tone
12. improvement in gait.

The aquatic therapist must be equipped with advanced knowledge and skill in the design of programs and in the application of interventions for patients. These applications fall under all areas of specialized medical and rehabilitative care including but not limited to orthopedics, sports medicine, neurology, cardiopulmonary medicine, acute care, pediatrics, and geriatrics. The aquatic therapist must have specialized training in aquatic therapy to implement aquatic therapy techniques but may hold an underlying credential in physical therapy, recreational therapy, or similar professional training.

The author, Dr. Luis Vargas, is recognized as an international expert in the field of aquatic therapy. Through his years of clinical experience Dr. Vargas developed the Diagnostic Aquatics Systems Integration (DASI) Theory that is used broadly today. This theory helped create a diagnostic evaluation instrument focusing on a systems approach that enables the aquatic therapist to formulate a functional diagnosis so that objectives can be established and a comprehensive aquatic rehabilitation plan of care can be designed and implemented. Diagnostic Aquatics Systems Integration is a therapeutic and diagnostic approach that provides a historical, empirical, and theoretical basis for the biomechanical, physiological, and neurophysiological principles and concepts that are the foundations of aquatic movement science. It is a systematic problem-solving approach that allows the trained aquatic therapist to make educated decisions and modifications to the techniques, activities, and interventions that are indicated for specific clinical problems.

Overview of Contents

This book provides the therapist with information about aquatic therapy and the specific techniques and protocols used in the delivery of therapy services using water and pools as part of the treatment modality.

The book is divided into three sections. Section I introduces the reader to the applied principles of using aquatic based interventions. It follows with the assessment process to decide if the patient is appropriate for aquatic therapy interventions and, if so, looks at how to decide on the types of interventions.

Section II provides information on specific intervention techniques including basic water-based therapy interventions and interventions based on specific styles including Bad Ragaz Ring Method, Watsu®, Halliwick, Clinical Wassertanzen, and Cardiaquatics.

Section III provides the therapist with information about diagnostic-specific concerns for patients with cardiopulmonary, neurologic, and musculoskeletal impairments.

The purpose of the book is to provide therapists with one reference that covers all the basic techniques used by aquatic therapists. As such it provides student therapists with an introduction to the various techniques used in aquatic therapy practice, clinically based therapists with a reference to help standardize treatment, and faculty members with a textbook that can be used as the primary book for classes in aquatic therapy.

Section I

Introduction to Aquatic Therapy

CHAPTER 1
APPLIED PRINCIPLES OF HYDRODYNAMICS

Historical Perspective

Since the dawn of time, hydrotherapy has been considered a valuable adjunct in the treatment of various musculoskeletal and neurologic disorders. Historically speaking, in ancient times the so-called Roman baths were used for relaxation purposes and to relieve common aches and pains. The thermal effects of the water were considered to be conducive to the relief of pain and enhancement of relaxation.

Likewise, the use of water for therapeutic purposes became a popular intervention in the clinical management of many orthopedic and neurological disorders. The rationale that supported the therapeutic application of hydrotherapy is attributed to the thermal effects of water on body tissues and on pain relief, as well as muscle relaxation, thereby having a positive effect on healing. The biophysical effects derived

from the use of hydrotherapy further support this premise.

Over the years, hydrotherapy has evolved into a new and rising specialty. Structured problem-oriented protocols and specialized clinical interventions have led to the emergence of aquatic therapy or aquatic rehabilitation. The past two decades have been pivotal to the development of this specialty. From the use of whirlpool tanks, which do not require active participation of the therapist, to the implementation of therapeutic pool protocols for a variety of diagnoses, aquatic therapists presently require specialized training in a number of clinical interventions that are unique to this specialty.

Physiological Effects

Hydrotherapy relies on the properties of water to provide a therapeutic environment that is superior to other possible environments and treatment modalities. The advantages of water include its ability to transfer heat effectively to a large part of the body and its use as a gentler means of applying physical stimuli or pressure to body parts and the body as a whole. Other properties that are important in hydrotherapy include buoyancy, hydrostatic pressure, cohesion, and viscosity. Let's look now at why these properties of water make it an excellent therapy medium.

Thermal Effects

Basically, the theory that explains the relief of pain and promotion of relaxation is rooted in the transfer of thermal energy. Thermal energy is transferred to the tissues by conduction and convection. Conduction is the transfer of energy from one medium, in this case water, to the other, which would be the skin. Convection refers to the widespread dissipation of this energy. Both means of thermal energy transfer could account for the success in the attainment of the already identified therapeutic goals. Comparatively, other thermotherapeutic modalities would limit this energy transfer to a smaller anatomical area.

In general, the therapeutic use of water can produce local or systemic biophysical effects that depend heavily on temperature and exposure. The higher the temperature, the more intense the effect. The larger the region exposed or treated, the greater the effect. Effects can be grouped into two categories. The first is temperature-based, dividing the effects into either thermotherapeutic or cryotherapeutic. The second divides them into systemic or localized. Systemically, cold water temperatures decrease the heart rate thereby decreasing the work of the myocardium and the cardiac output. When this happens, blood pressure increases due to an increase in peripheral vascular resistance as a result of induced vasoconstriction. Conversely, warm water temperatures cause vasodilation. This is an important consideration when our goal is to improve circulation. In addition to the direct impact that increased water temperature has on vasomotor tone, effects on muscle tone have been identified. Hypertonicity is affected under the same condition by a decrease in muscle tone.

According to Lehman, the temperature range of the water must fall within 92°F to 96°F in order for therapeutic value to be attained. If the water temperature falls below the lowest established value, no significant therapeutic effect will result. Conversely, if it significantly exceeds this range, tissue damage can occur. The exception to this rule is the person with multiple sclerosis, based on the premise that heat triggers the clinical manifestations that are characteristic of this neurological disorder. For people with multiple sclerosis lower water temperature ranging from 88°F to 90°F is considered more beneficial.

Heat inhibits the firing of the type II afferent intrafusal fibers of the muscle spindle supplying the agonist. These fibers are also referred to as alpha motor neurons. Increased and uncontrolled hyperactivity of these fibers due to a stretch of the muscle spindle causes a sustained tonic extrafusal fiber involuntary contraction leading to the development of a muscle spasm (Figure 1). Inhibition of these fibers occurs when the Golgi tendon organ of the nerve ending is activated in the antagonist. The result is a decrease in spasmodic activity thereby breaking up the

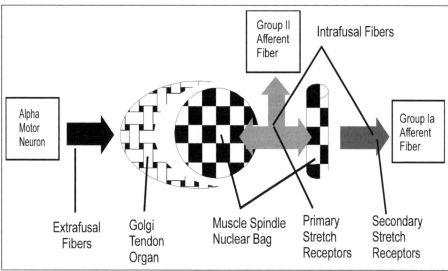

Figure 1: The muscle spindle involved in muscle spasms, showing the type Ia and type II afferent intrafusal stretch receptors and the extrafusal alpha motor neuron supplying the Golgi tendon organ.

spasm-pain-spasm cycle. This is the same premise that explains reduction of muscle tone in the presence of spasticity.

The neuromuscular effects of thermal aquatic therapy on pain relief are not only attributed to alterations in muscle spindle hyperactivity but additionally to alterations in nerve conduction velocity. The application of heat over the area of a peripheral nerve raises the pain threshold of that nerve.

The viscoelastic properties of connective tissue are also affected beneficially when exposed to increases in water temperature by restoring elasticity and plastic deformation properties.

Thermal hydrotherapy is particularly beneficial in addressing inflammation. While aquatic therapy can offer many advantages in acute inflammatory disorders depending on water temperature, caution should be taken in these cases not to cause an increase in joint effusion and edema by integrating activities that might promote a significant increase in circulation to the affected joints.

Mechanical Effects

The hydrotherapeutic use of tanks and mechanical turbines produces a turbulent whirlpool effect on the tissues in the form of a hydromassage. This hydromassage is of clinical value in reducing localized spasmodic activity, in reducing pain, in improving circulation, and in promoting new granulation tissue and blunt debridement of necrotic eschar tissue in burns and open wounds.

Properties of Water and Applied Physics

There are four identified biophysical properties of water. These properties are applied therapeutically to attain clinical goals and objectives. Facilitation or inhibition of motor function depends on the appropriate implementation of these properties in activities or interventions that are part of the plan of care. The four properties of water are buoyancy, hydrostatic pressure, viscosity, and cohesion.

Buoyancy and the Principle of Archimedes

The first of these properties is called buoyancy. When a body is immersed in water, it experiences an upward thrust that is equal to its weight (Figure 2). This law of physics explains the property of buoyancy and is known as Archimedes' principle. As gravity decreases secondary to the effects of buoyancy, the weight-bearing forces acting upon a joint will also decrease. Consequently, the body is rendered weightless. Weightlessness allows a reduction in joint compression forces. When the forces that act upon a joint

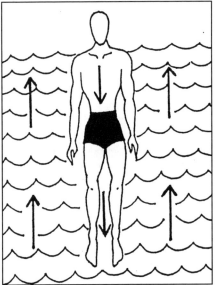

Figure 2: The principle of Archimedes and the property of buoyancy. Buoyancy in water gives the experience of an upward thrust.

are relieved, the result is increased pain-free mobility or decreased pain levels. This explains the effect of buoyancy on pain relief. Patients will be able to perform pain-free activities or at least activities with lower levels of pain.

Buoyancy can also be used to challenge patients with postural deficits who experience difficulty in maintaining a fixed or aligned position in shallow or deep water. Consequently, buoyancy is also beneficial in challenging postural alignment.

When applying the laws of physics to a buoyant body, it is important to consider the concept of relative density. Whether a body sinks or floats in water depends on its relative density. The relative density of water equals 1.0. If a body's density is less than 1.0, the body tends to float. If it is greater, the body will sink. When we take a deep breath before immersing ourselves under water, our relative density will decrease. Therefore, our body will have a tendency to float. The opposite will happen when we exhale before or during an immersion under water.

Relative density differs depending on gender. Males have an average relative density of .95 while the average relative density of females is .75.

Hydrostatic Pressure and Pascal's Law

Pascal's law indicates that when a body is immersed in water there is a pressure exerted by the fluid upon the tissues. This is referred to as hydrostatic pressure and is the second property of water (Figure 3). The degree of hydrostatic pressure that is exerted upon the tissues depends on two factors, the density of the fluid and the depth of immersion. When fluid density

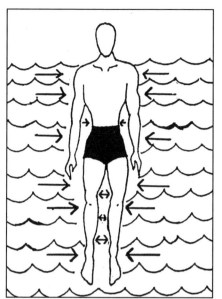

Figure 3: Pascal's law states that depth and density influence the hydrostatic pressure exerted upon the tissues.

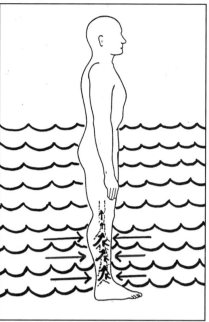

Figure 4: The effect of hydrostatic pressure on venous circulation.

increases, so does hydrostatic pressure. For instance, seawater has a higher density than fresh water. Consequently, the effects of hydrostatic pressure will be greater in the ocean than in a swimming pool.

When water depth is at shoulder level, the hydrostatic pressure experienced is twice as high as that experienced when water depth is at hip level. The latter example can be used as an applied clinical objective to prevent venous stasis in cases of venous insufficiency (Figure 4). As a property of water, hydrostatic pressure can also be clinically applied in the reeducation of breathing patterns for patients with weak primary respiratory musculature.

Furthermore, when the thorax is immersed in water to the shoulder level, the hydrostatic pressure exerted will assist the vital capacity while at the same time resisting inspiratory capacity (Figure 5). This effect will result in

strengthening the diaphragm and intercostal muscles. These patients might experience dyspnea and anxiety as a result of their inability to maintain

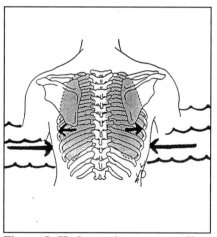

Figure 5: Hydrostatic pressure affects vital capacity and tidal volume by strengthening primary respiratory muscles.

adequate ventilation due to the effects of hydrostatic pressure on the weak muscular structures, especially if they rely on the use of the accessory muscles of respiration.

Another effective clinical application of hydrostatic pressure is the stimulation of sensory input that occurs as the density of the fluid exerts pressure upon the tissues. It refers to the tactile effect generated by this pressure. This might be a beneficial consideration for patients with sensory deficits resulting from neuropathies.

Both buoyancy and hydrostatic pressure interact together to produce the weightlessness effects and the applied consequences of these effects.

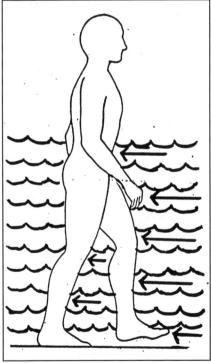

Figure 6: Friction produced by liquid resists the movement of a body, thereby strengthening soft tissues.

Viscosity, Cohesion, and the Application of Bernoulli's Law

Bernoulli's law addresses the last two properties of water, viscosity and cohesion. Cohesion is the gathering of molecules to form a liquid. Viscosity refers to the density of the liquid and its effects on the surface of a body as it moves through the liquid.

When our primary objective is to strengthen weak muscles, the property responsible for the attainment of this outcome is viscosity. When a body moves in water, friction is produced between the body and the water (Figure 6). This friction resists the movement of the body through the water. This resistance produces a strengthening effect on soft tissues. Bernoulli's law establishes a relationship between the fluid friction and the velocity of movement. Consequently, hydrodynamic forces play an important role in this applied law of aquatic physics.

Hydrodynamically speaking, when a body moves through the water, the friction exerted by the water produces a stronger resistance in front of the moving body than it does posteriorly. If the body is moving against a turbulent flow as opposed to a streamlined or steady flow, the resistance will be higher. When this happens, a series of wave-like circular patterns called eddies will be evident behind the moving body (Figure 7).

As the pressure decreases behind the moving body, a drag force known as a wake is produced. The faster the body moves through the water the greater the drag force. Consequently, a larger wake means that a greater resistance is being experienced. This principle is useful in the application of balance training and postural awareness activities performed in shallow water.

Patients with balance problems and postural deficits will have a tendency to experience more difficulty with forward gait and retrogait activities in shallow water while observing postural alignment.

Bougier's Theorem and the Concept of the Metacenter

The metacenter is the center of buoyancy. Anatomically the center of buoyancy is located at T11 (Figure 8). When the metacenter is directly above the center of gravity located at S2, the body is in a state of equilibrium in the water. This state of equilibrium will determine the stability of the body in

the water. This theory is known as Bougier's Theorem.

The concept of the metacenter is used to explain the lack of equilibrium that patients with hemiplegia or amputations experience in the water. In the supine position, patients who have limitations as a result of a stroke will have a tendency to roll towards the spastic or affected side secondary to a shift in the alignment between the center of buoyancy and the center of gravity. The same is true with individuals who have had an amputation. Conversely, a patient who presents with an edematous extremity will roll away from the affected limb for the same reason, a shift in the alignment of both centers. If both centers are malaligned,

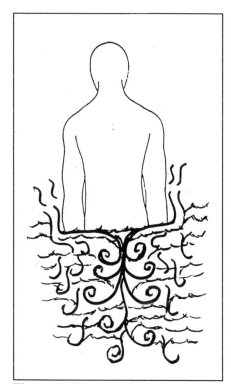

Figure 7: The circular waves called eddies formed as a body moves forward through the water produce a drag force posterior to the body.

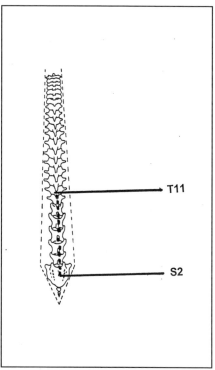

Figure 8: The alignment of the center of buoyancy (T11) and the center of gravity (S2) as described in Bougier's Theorem.

maintaining a vertical position for deep-water activities while wearing floatation gear will be difficult. The patient will have a tendency to fall forward or backward in deep water. How, then, can we bring about a proper alignment? The response lies in the position or movement of the head and upper extremities in relation to the trunk or the affected limb.

Applied Halliwick techniques or the applied facilitation of brainstem level reflexes in selected neurological cases might be effective strategies in realigning the metacenter with the center of gravity. These interventions will be explained in Chapter 5.

Conclusion

The success in the attainment of treatment goals and functional outcomes in aquatic therapy are partially attributed to the properties of water, the applied laws of physics supporting each property, and the physiologic effects derived from the application of specialized interventions, activities, and protocols.

CHAPTER 2
THE DIAGNOSTIC AQUATICS SYSTEMS INTEGRATION THEORY

In order to identify the pertinent clinical problems, establish functional goals and objectives, and design an aquatic rehabilitation plan of care that would address the identified problems, a comprehensive, initial pre-aquatic evaluation must be done upon patient referral.

The Diagnostic Aquatics Systems Integration (DASI) Approach features a land-based systems assessment that evaluates performance and function with emphasis on specific tests and measurements (Appendix 1). This land-based systems assessment contains several fundamental components: musculoskeletal, cardiopulmonary, neurological, and functional.

Prior to the evaluation, the patient should be invited for a tour of the facility, which will give him the opportunity to briefly observe a pool session with other patients being treated. The patient should sign a Con-sent for Treatment form in addition to all other health insurance forms as required by the clinic. Many facilities produce an orientation videotape for the patient to watch prior to the evaluation and first treatment.

The patient evaluation should take place in a designated evaluation room at the clinic where the pool is located. At the time of the initial pre-aquatic evaluation, the patient should be dressed in a bathing suit. This will allow the therapist to identify with accuracy, through visual and surface anatomy examination, any postural deviations, evidence of spasmodic activity, trigger points of pain, gait deviations, edema, dyskinesia and weakness, sensory deficits, or limitations in range of motion. No shoes should be worn to allow an accurate gait analysis. The patient should receive a detailed explanation of all the components of the diagnostic assessment. The evaluation is designed to last from one to one and a half hours.

Medical History

The first step for the therapist in the DASI Pre-Aquatic Evaluation will be to record the patient's history. If the referral is unclear as to the patient's diagnosis, the therapist should clarify any questions with the referring physician prior to the patient's appointment. The recorded history must include the clinical problem or diagnosis and how the problem occurred, reported symptoms and signs, associated medical or surgical problems, and medications taken by the patient. Any precautions or contraindications should also be recorded.

Musculoskeletal Assessment

Manual Muscle Test and Goniometry

The musculoskeletal component assesses strength, joint range, joint edema, spasmodic activity, posture, and leg-length discrepancy. An integrated manual muscle test with a goniometric evaluation is the first part of the assessment. All major joints are tested for range of motion and muscle strength including the spine at all levels. When goniometrically evaluating the spine, two instruments are highly recommended. These are the CROM (cervical range of motion) instrument (Figure 9) and the BROM (back range of motion) instrument. The BROM is used to measure lumbar range of motion. However, the use of an inclinometer is also highly suggested if the other instruments are not available (Figure 10). Measurement of the extremity joints can be accomplished using the

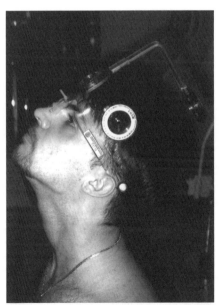

Figure 9: Measurement of cervical extension using the CROM.

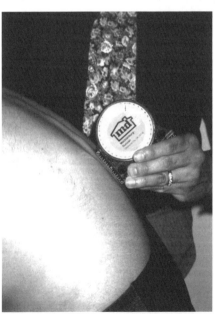

Figure 10: Measurement of lumbar function using an inclinometer.

conventional goniometer (Figure 11). Muscle groups are targeted in the manual muscle test as opposed to isolated muscle testing (Figure 12).

Inspection is another fundamental element in the DASI Pre-Aquatic Evaluation. The degree of active or passive movement, whether pain free or painful must be assessed prior to recording any measurements.

Inspection will be the first evidence suggesting restrictions in range of motion or muscle weakness. If the patient complains of pain through the range but demonstrates functional range of motion, this is referred to as kinemyalgia (muscular pain upon active movement). It could be found in a muscle or a group of muscles and can be further rated using the Visual Analog Scale or the Numeric Pain Scale.

If the patient experiences articular pain during active or passive movement through the arc of motion, this is called

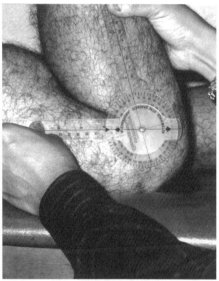

Figure 11: Measurement of knee flexion using a conventional goniometer.

kinearthralgia. Furthermore, assessment of skin color in the affected region for evidence of erythema, ecchymoses,

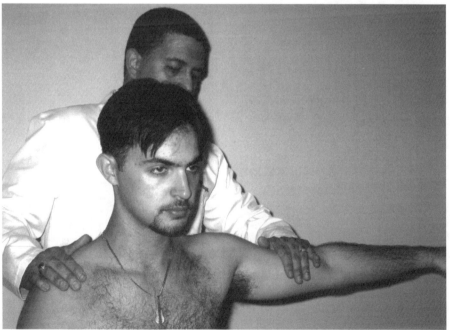

Figure 12: Manual muscle testing of the shoulder abductors.

cyanosis, or a hematoma is also an important consideration when inspecting the area.

Evaluation of Girth

If there is edema, girth measurements are taken in order to identify evidence of edema and establish differences between extremities (Figure 13). The routine procedure consists of identifying an anatomical landmark at which point the measurement is taken with a tape measure.

Assessment of Leg Length

In cases involving the lower extremities, it is important to consider leg-length discrepancy, as this will have an impact on gait. The conventional test uses a simple tape measure with two anatomical landmarks as references: the ASIS (anterior superior iliac spine) and the lateral malleolus (Figure 14). A

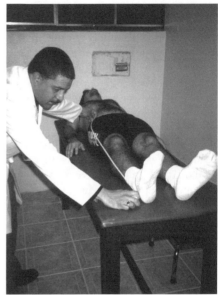

Figure 14: Measurement of leg length to determine discrepancy.

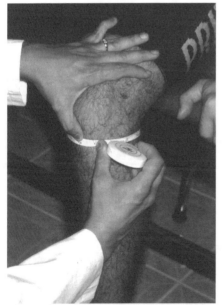

Figure 13: Girth measurement of the knee to determine edema using the patellar apex as a landmark.

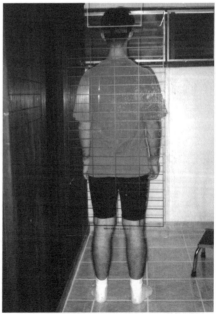

Figure 15: Assessing posture in the coronal plane.

contralateral comparison of the measurements will determine if there is a leg-length discrepancy.

Patients with a history of fractures and surgery to the lower extremities, particularly the hips, will very likely present evidence of leg-length discrepancy.

Posture Assessment

A routine posture assessment where deviations are identified in the coronal and sagittal planes as well as both the anterior and posterior views should follow this (Figure 15 and Figure 16).

Posture assessment is part of the inspection because we are focusing on a visual examination with surface anatomy applications. The pathway of the line of gravity should be used as reference for the identification of postural deviations during this assessment (Figure 17).

In the evaluation of posture, the therapist must inspect the alignment of the spine, including the head, in relation to the line of gravity for both sagittal and coronal views. Lateral, forward, and axial displacements should be recorded accordingly. Additional appendicular displacements such as excessive anterior or posterior pelvic rotation should also be noted (Figure 18).

Evaluation of Spasmodic Activity

Following the posture assessment, a surface anatomy examination to determine evidence of spasmodic

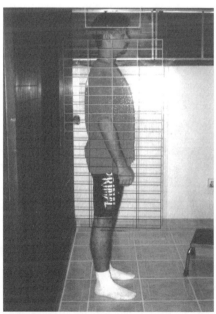

Figure 16: Assessing posture in the sagittal plane.

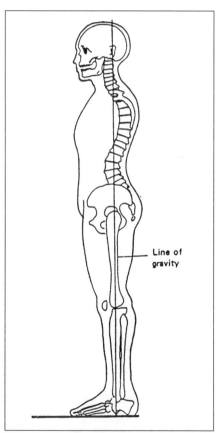

Line of gravity

Figure 17: Graphic illustration of the line of gravity used as reference in a posture assessment.

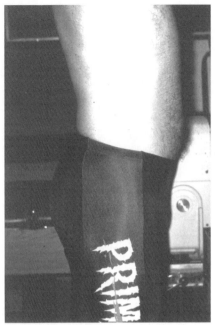

Figure 18: Anterior pelvic rotation as seen in a sagittal view.

activity or soft tissue tightness should be performed using the Spasmodic Activity Grading (SAG) Scale.

Table 1: Grades of Spasms

Grade 1 = a single nodular spasm, approximately 1-2 cm. circumference.

Grade 2 = multinodular, more than two spasmodic nodules in a single muscle.

Grade 3 = widespread nodular, multiple spasmodic nodules in more than one muscle.

Grade 4 = widespread anodular, no defined nodules palpated but instead excessive tension is palpated with tenderness present throughout one or more muscles.

Palpation is the fundamental technique used in this examination. Emphasis should be placed on palpation of the affected area or areas but a generalized surface anatomy examination is advised because problems in other regions that have not been reported in diagnosis or history can be identified.

Comprehensive knowledge and

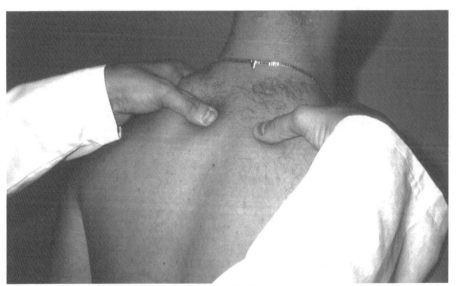

Figure 19: Evaluating for spasmodic activity and active trigger points in the scapular region using surface anatomy techniques.

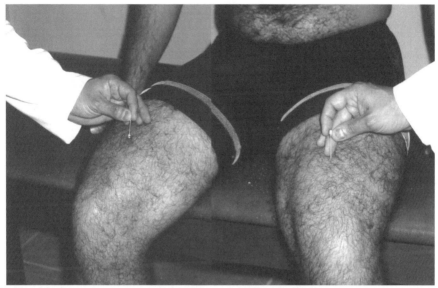

Figure 20: Sensory assessment for sharp-dull discrimination.

skill covering surface anatomy, gross anatomy, neuroanatomy, and kinesiology are essential in order to competently perform this examination. Bony landmarks are palpated as reference points for the accurate evaluation of soft tissues. Additionally, the therapist should isolate muscles in order to adequately identify any soft tissue problems. See Table 1.

The surface anatomy examination integrates the trigger point test, which is used to detect tenderness at the spasmodic site. As the examiner is palpating soft tissues, he runs the palmar surface of the thumb along the anatomical region (Figure 19). In muscles, this technique is applied with

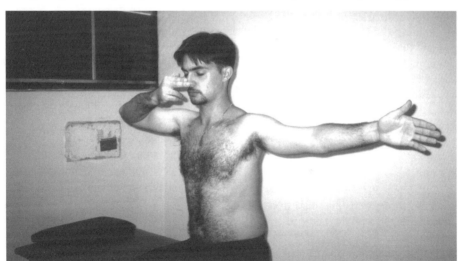

Figure 21: The finger-to-nose test is used to determine intact upper extremity coordination.

considerable pressure from origin to insertion. When the patient identifies pain, the examiner stops at the exact site. If a muscle spasm is identified, the trigger point test will be positive at that site. The Numeric Pain Scale or the more complicated McGill Pain Scale can be used to grade the level of tenderness. The Numeric Pain Scale is utilized in the neurological component of the DASI Pre-Aquatic Evaluation to assess the intensity and severity of pain (Appendix 1).

Neurological Assessment

Superficial Sensation and Coordination

The first function to be tested in the neurological assessment is superficial sensation. The two-point discrimination and the sharp-dull discrimination tests (Figure 20) are used for this purpose. A basic test for static and dynamic coordination is performed in this component of the DASI evaluation. Dynamic coordination of the upper extremities should be tested (Figure 21). Lower extremity dynamic coordination can be evaluated by having the patient perform a tandem gait test (Figure 22) or a simple walk test. Likewise, static coordination and balance can be tested with Romberg's test.

Proprioception

The alpha motor neurons or type I fibers of the muscle spindle supplying the Golgi tendon organ (GTO) influence proprioception.

Proprioception is the sense of position of the parts of the body in space. Testing for an intact proprioceptive ability involves having the patient identify the position of an extremity,

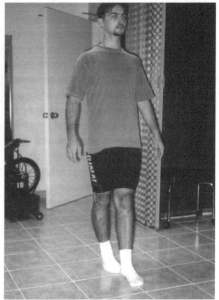

Figure 22: The tandem gait test is used to determine lower extremity coordination.

joint, or body part with the eyes closed. The examiner moves the extremity or body part passively in order for the patient to describe its position in space (Figure 23).

Deep Tendon Reflexes

Evaluation of the myotatic reflexes in order to determine reflex arc pathology is another neurological test. The reflex arc involves a sensory and a motor neuron. Upon stimulation, the receptor transmits the impulse through the sensory or afferent neuron to the central nervous system where it synapses with an interneuron. The impulse is then transmitted to the motor or efferent neuron and onto the effector organ, which is the muscle (Figure 24).

Two myotatic reflexes are tested in the DASI Pre-Aquatic Evaluation. These are the biceps reflex and the patellar reflex or knee jerk (Figure 25). When the biceps and patellar tendons

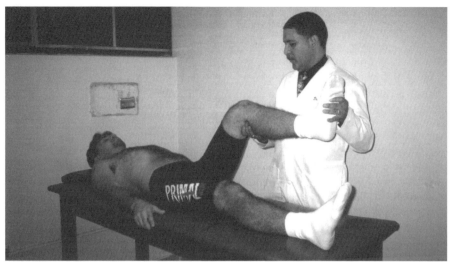

Figure 23: The examiner passively flexes the knee with the patient's eyes closed to test for lower extremity proprioception.

are tapped, the response is a quick jerk. The absence of a response as well as evidence of hyperreflexia or hypore-flexia would suggest pathology.

Balance

Intact balance or lack thereof can be assessed by performing the same tests used to evaluate coordination.

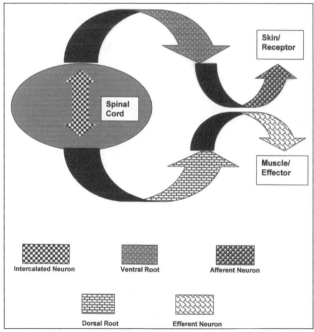

Figure 24: Graphic illustration of the reflex arc.

These have been discussed earlier in the neurological assessment and are mainly concerned with dynamic balance. When evaluating static balance, the patient is sitting at the edge of the examination table with the arms at 90° shoulder abduction (Figure 26). The examiner challenges the patient's balance in this position by pushing slightly in all directions. If the patient's static balance is affected, he will not be able to maintain this position and will attempt to use the arms to prevent falling. Romberg's test can also be used to assess static balance. Evidence of impaired balance might suggest vestibular problems.

Pain

Part of the evaluation of pain was discussed earlier in the musculoskeletal assessment. The Diagnostic Aquatic Systems Integration approach utilizes the Numeric Pain Scale to grade the

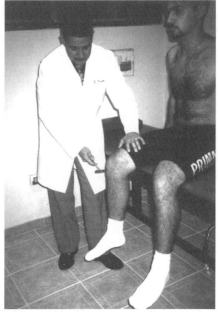

Figure 25: Testing patellar tendon reflexes.

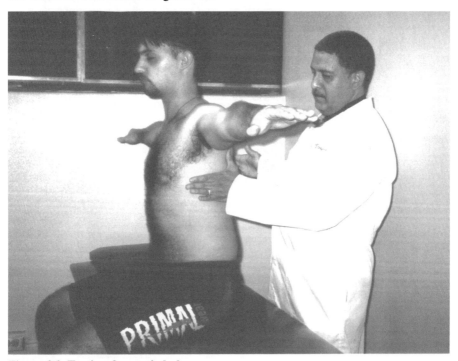

Figure 26: Testing for static balance.

patient's interpretation of pain. However, the McGill Pain Scale, which is more comprehensive and lengthy, can also be used. Likewise, the trigger point test is useful in detecting localized pain and tenderness. When we measure pain, we must consider the subjective nature of this assessment. Some patients have a higher pain threshold and tolerance than others. Therefore, what one patient might describe as level 3 pain another patient might identify as level 8. It is important for the examiner to further correlate the patient's reported level of pain and the impact on functional activities. This will provide the examiner with a more accurate clinical picture of the problem.

Muscle Tone

When the examiner moves a joint passively with the patient relaxed in a supine position, the joint should not present any resistance to the movement. In patients suffering from neurological disorders, there will be a certain level of involuntary resistance to the passive motion. This indicates hypertonicity or spasticity, which is defined as a state of continuous mild to severe contraction of a muscle. Upon palpation, the muscle feels similar to a muscle with grade 4 spasmodic activity; that is, the entire muscle feels considerably tight and bulky. The difference lies in the fact that spasticity is a central nervous system problem affecting the extrapyramidal pathways while a muscle spasm involves a localized reaction of the myofibril to a stretch of the muscle spindle.

Hypotonicity or significantly decreased tone is a clinical problem present in patients with flaccid paraly-

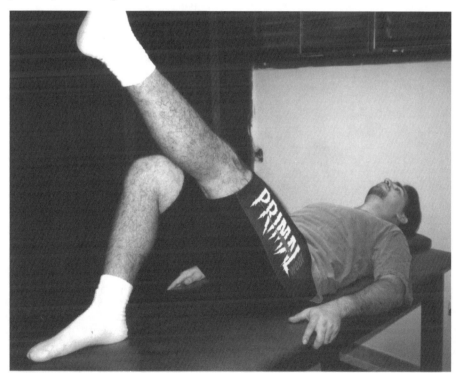

Figure 27: The straight-leg raise test to locate the point of pain in the back.

sis. Hypotonic muscles feel soft and flabby upon palpation. Consequently, when passively ranged, the extremity might appear hypermobile. This is characteristic of patients in the acute stage of spinal cord injury or stroke.

Cogwheel rigidity is a clinical sign found in patients with parkinsonian characteristics. It is characterized by involuntary jerky movements of the passively ranged extremity throughout the full arc of motion.

Muscle contractures can occur as a result of changes in the elastic deformation properties of connective and soft tissue. Severely hypertonic muscles can further influence the development of a contracture. When a contracture is present, the joint or joints involved are fixed with severe restrictions in range of motion and tightening of the affected tendons. Passive motion is, therefore, not possible.

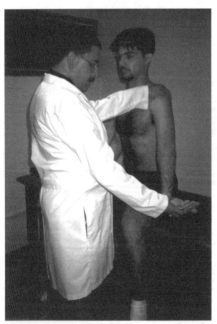

Figure 28: Neural tension test for the radial nerve.

Problem-Specific Neurological Tests

Straight Leg Raise Test

For this test, the patient is positioned supine with one leg flexed and the other extended on the table. Maintaining the knee extended, the patient is asked to raise the affected extremity to the point of pain (Figure 27). The examiner should note the exact measurement or point when the pain begins. This test will be positive in patients suffering from low back pain associated with disc herniations, sciatica, piriformis syndrome, or lumbar radiculopathy. The reported pain might be localized to the low back region where the problem exists or it might radiate to the posterior aspect of the affected lower extremity. It might be unilateral or bilateral.

Neural Tension Tests

The neural tension tests determine involvement of three nerves supplying the upper extremity. These are the ulnar, radial, and median nerves. If these tests are positive, the problems might be peripheral or radicular in nature. Radicular involvement suggests problems in the brachial plexus at any of the segments that participate in the formation of the nerve. Pain radiating throughout the upper extremity following the distribution of the nerve would render the test positive. The reported pain might begin proximally in the cervical region. If this were the case, it would suggest brachial plexus involvement as opposed to a peripheral problem.

1. Radial Nerve — this test is performed with the patient sitting at the edge of the examination table or standing. The examiner pas-

sively depresses the shoulder with the elbow fully extended. The patient is asked to internally rotate the upper extremity and flex the wrist. The arm is positioned at the side. The therapist then performs a series of oscillating and alternating abduction and adduction short arc movements of the shoulder (Figure 28).

2. Median Nerve — this test is performed using the same procedure and position of the upper extremity described in the radial nerve test. However, the patient is asked to externally rotate the upper extremity and extend the wrist fully (Figure 29).

3. Ulnar Nerve — the patient is seated or standing for this test and is asked to externally rotate the upper extremity with the arm at 90° of abduction and the wrist fully extended (Figure 30).

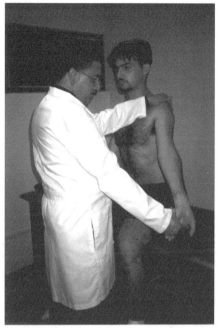

Figure 29: Neural tension test for the median nerve.

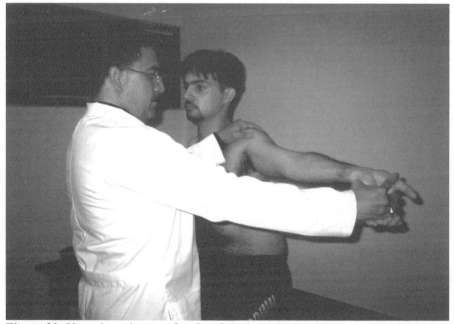

Figure 30: Neural tension test for the ulnar nerve.

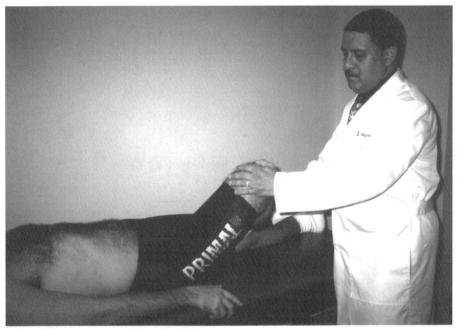

Figure 31: Testing for Fabere sign.

Fabere Sign

The Fabere Sign (also called Patrick's Sign) is a popular test used to identify sciatica secondary to piriformis syndrome. A positive Fabere sign might also indicate disc disease with radiculopathy. The patient is positioned supine with one extremity fully extended. The opposite or involved extremity is flexed at the knee and the heel of the foot is placed against the extended knee (Figure 31). The patient is then asked to externally rotate that same hip. If pain is elicited, this would render the test positive.

Cervical Compression Test

Patients diagnosed with cervical radiculopathy will experience an increase in the intensity and onset of symptoms when this test is performed. The patient is seated. The therapist rests both elbows near the acromioclavicular joint with both hands clasped at the top of the patient's head (Figure 32). The patient's head is aligned passively in

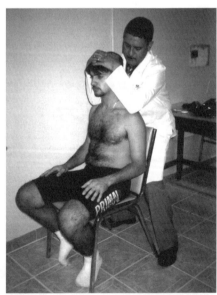

Figure 32: The cervical compression test.

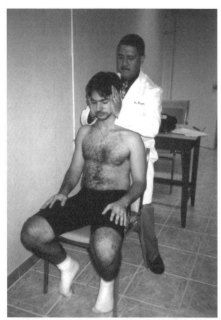

Figure 33: The cervical distraction stretch test.

axial extension as the examiner exerts compression in a caudal direction.

Distraction-Stretch Test

The DASI approach implements this test and defines it as a supplement to the compression test. If the compression test is positive, cervical distraction would then decrease the symptoms and signs resulting in a radicular release of pressure. Cervical distraction is performed in a sitting or supine position with emphasis on a unilateral stretch followed by a bilateral stretch (Figure 33). The cervical spine should be positioned in axial extension for a more effective stretch.

Vertebral Artery Test

The patient is in the supine position with his head out of the superior edge of the table and held by the examiner's hand at the occiput. The therapist flexes, laterally flexes, and rotates the patient's head and neck in both directions with the patient's eyes open, checking for pupil dilation and other clinical signs such as lightheadedness (Figure 34). These signs would indicate

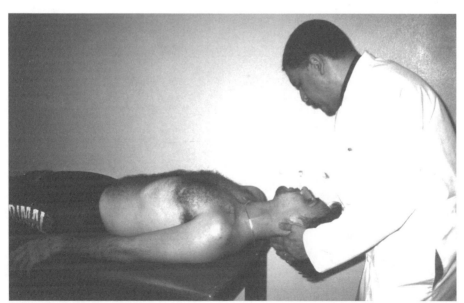

Figure 34: The vertebral artery test.

involvement of the vertebral artery, which is a clinical finding in patients with cervical spine injuries and associated radiculopathies.

the apex of the dens of the axis and attaches laterally on each side at the internal border of the foramen magnum. Its function is to restrict excessive rotation and lateral flexion of the neck in each direction. Changes in the viscoelastic properties of this ligament

Alar Ligament Test

The alar ligament emerges from

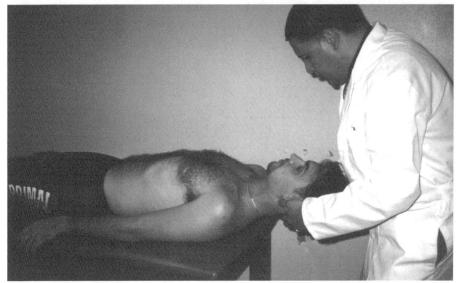

Figure 35: The alar ligament test, starting position.

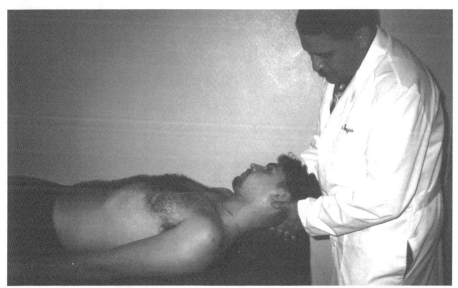

Figure 36: The alar ligament test, rotating the cervical spine.

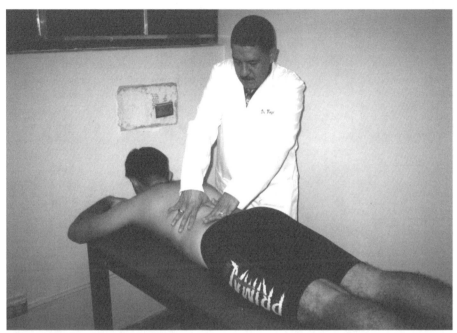

Figure 37: The vertebral glide test.

will not only reveal limitations in cervical rotation but can also further influence cervical pain and the onset of migraines and headaches. With the patient supine, the head and neck are positioned in axial extension. The examiner holds the patient's head at the occiput. The therapist performs rotation of the cervical spine in both directions and checks for restrictions in movement and the onset of pain (Figure 35 and Figure 36).

Vertebral Glide Test

This test is performed to rule out the onset of localized or radiated pain in either the upper or lower extremities with or without numbness when vertebra glides on vertebra in an anterior direction. Therefore, it applies to the cervical or lumbar parts of the spine because their spinous processes are oriented horizontally. The patient is prone. The therapist exerts gentle pressure on the spinous processes of each cervical or lumbar vertebra mobilizing the vertebra in a posteroanterior direction (Figure 37).

Babinski Sign

The Babinski sign is a maneuver that evaluates the integrity of extensor plantar reflexes. With the sharp end of

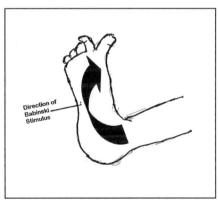

Figure 38: Graphic illustration of the Babinski sign.

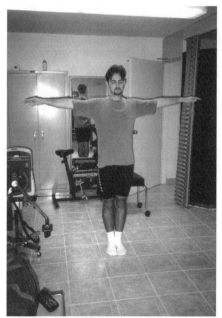

Figure 39: Romberg's test for balance.

the reflex hammer, the examiner strokes the plantar surface of the patient's foot (Figure 38). The stimulus begins at the calcaneus and moves medially towards the great toe. A positive response will elicit extension of the great toe with fanning of the four lateral toes. A positive Babinski is associated with neuropathology in children and adults.

Romberg's Test

The patient stands with his feet close together and his eyes closed. The arms could be at his sides or abducted at 90° (Figure 39). If the patient sways to either side, it would indicate a positive response. This balance impairment would further suggest cerebellar or vestibular problems.

The neurological tests described in this section are important tools in the differential diagnosis of problem-specific peripheral and central nervous system disorders. However, other neurological exams can be performed depending on the patient's diagnosis and the clinical judgment of the therapist. Should that be the case, any additional test must be documented accordingly in the DASI Pre-Aquatic Evaluation Form. The selection of one or more of the tests featured in the DASI evaluation strictly depends on the patient's diagnosis and medical history. For instance, if the patient is referred with a cervical radiculopathy diagnosis, the following tests might assist the clinician in establishing a differential functional diagnosis:

1. Neural Tension Tests
2. Cervical Compression Test
3. Distraction Stretch Test
4. Vertebral Artery Test
5. Vertebral Glide Test
6. Alar Ligament Test

Cardiopulmonary Assessment

Recording the respiratory rate is a routine technique in the cardiopulmonary component of the DASI evaluation. An increased respiratory rate would suggest the presence of dyspnea or tachypnea. The examiner would further be able to determine evidence of respiratory distress with recruitment of the accessory respiratory muscles. The most commonly hyperactive accessory muscles are the sternocleidomastoid and the scalenes.

The Diagnostic Aquatics Systems Integration approach to the pre-aquatic assessment describes three pulmonary evaluation techniques that are performed in an effort to assess respiratory function. These are thoracic auscultation, mediate percussion, and evaluation of thoracic symmetry.

Thoracic Auscultation

Thoracic auscultation features the examination of pulmonary and cardiac sounds. Auscultation of the lungs is performed on the seated patient by using the diaphragm of the stethoscope (Figure 40). The objective is to determine the presence of normal, abnormal, or adventitious breath sounds. As a routine procedure, pulmonary auscultation should be performed during the pre-aquatic assessment. However, it will be of significant clinical value if the patient presents with a history of primary or secondary pulmonary problems.

The presence of normal breath sounds would rule out evidence of tracheobronchial secretions or pathology in the lung parenchyma. Depending on the pattern heard on auscultation, normal breath sounds are either vesicular or bronchovesicular and would provide clinical evidence that the lungs are cleared of exudate, secretions, or interstitial pathology. However, abnormal and adventitious breath sounds would indicate pulmonary histopathology, which may be associated with malignancy or with a viral, bacterial, or fungal infection. Abnormal breath sounds can be grouped as bronchial, diminished, or absent and would indicate the presence of an underlying

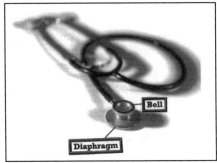

Figure 40: The bell and diaphragm of a stethoscope.

solid, liquid, or gas medium that interferes with the normal transmission of breath sounds. Adventitious breath sounds point towards the presence of secretions in the airway secondary to intrapulmonary infections or malignancy.

The patient's social history should be taken into consideration when completing a pulmonary assessment. Associated risks should be identified. For instance, smokers tend to develop characteristic rales and a typical cough. This would have an impact on the patient's endurance to aquatic physical activities causing early distress and decreased tolerance.

Pulmonary auscultation should be performed with the patient sitting (Figure 41). The suggested sequence is apex to base. The examiner should auscultate all segments and lobes bilaterally in order to compare both sides.

Recording the patient's heart rate and blood pressure should be the first step in the assessment of cardiovascular function. The heart contracts on systole and refills on diastole. The heart produces two normal sounds when the myocardium contracts. These sounds are caused by the opening and closing of the atrioventricular and semilunar valves. We commonly refer to them as the lubb-dubb of the heart. But clinically, they are referred to as S1 and S2 respectively. Three positions are described for cardiac auscultation: sitting (the most common), supine, and left-lateral recumbent. These positions allow the borders or areas of the heart to move closer to the thoracic wall to allow a more accurate auscultation. Cardiac auscultation is performed with the bell of the stethoscope (Figure 40). Four anatomical areas are used as

referenced landmarks for cardiac auscultation (Figure 42):
1. left lateral sternal border (LLSB), which is anatomically located at the fourth intercostal space to the left of the sternum.

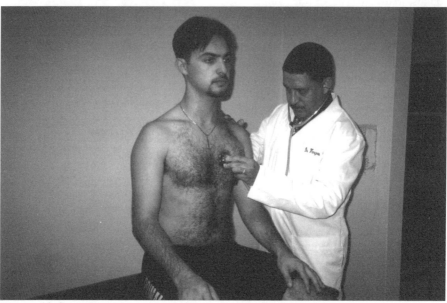

Figure 41: The therapist performs auscultation of the lungs.

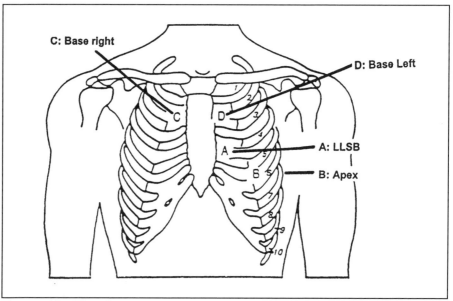

Figure 42: The four anatomical areas used as landmarks for cardiac auscultation.

2. apex, which is anatomically located at the fifth intercostal space to left of the sternum.

3. base right, which is anatomically located at the second intercostal space to the right of the sternum and is known as the pulmonic area.

4. base left, which is anatomically located at the second intercostal space to the left of the sternum and is known as the aortic area.

Heard over the LLSB, S1 is associated with closure of the atrioventricular valves. When these valves do not close simultaneously, the sound can be heard separately and is then called a split. Uneven timing of mitral and tricuspid valve closure causes a split. S2 marks closure of the semilunar valves and is heard over base right for the pulmonic valve and base left for the aortic valve. A physiologic split of S2 can also occur and is considered normal.

The pathologic cardiac sounds are S3 and S4. Heard at the apex or LLSB. S3 is a distinctive sound that follows S2 and is known as a ventricular gallop. When heard, it may indicate coronary artery disease, cardiomyopathy, or valvular disease. S3 is characteristically the first sign of congestive heart failure. The fourth cardiac sound (S4) precedes S1 and is called an atrial gallop. This sound is also heard at the apex or at the LLSB and is a clinical sign in patients with atrial fibrillation.

Other pathologic cardiac sounds include murmurs and ejection clicks. Murmurs are sustained abnormal vibrations of the heart valves. They are a characteristic clinical finding in patients with rheumatic valve disease. Ejection clicks are usually isolated sounds related to a dysfunction of the aortic or pulmonic valves, or to a ballooning of one of the cusps of the mitral valve.

Mediate Percussion

The second pulmonary assessment technique is called mediate percussion. The examiner identifies the intercostal space, places the palmar surface of the middle finger in each space, and then taps the nail of that finger with the

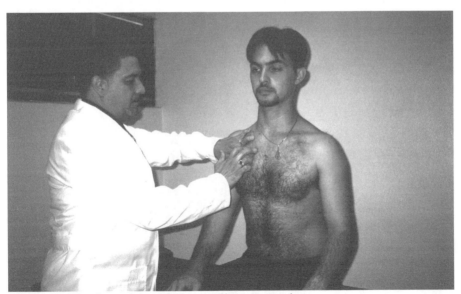

Figure 43: The therapist performs mediate percussion.

index or middle fingers of the opposite hand (Figure 43) evoking a characteristic sound called resonance. The normal finding is a resonant chest. If the sound obtained is dull, flat, or excessively high-pitched, it might suggest the presence of a solid, liquid, or air medium in the chest cavity interfering with sound conduction.

Thoracic Symmetry

The evaluation of thoracic symmetry will determine the extent and strength of thoracic excursions, thereby assessing the function of the intercostal muscles and diaphragm. This test can be performed from an anterior or a posterior approach. If the anterior

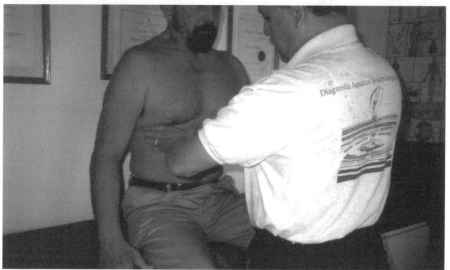

Figure 44: The anterior approach used to measure thoracic symmetry.

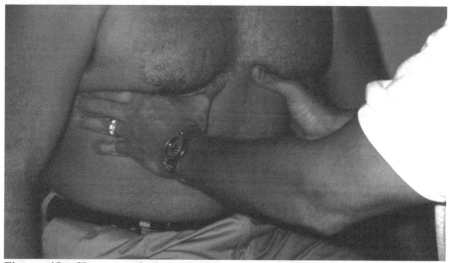

Figure 45: Close-up of the anterior approach used to measure thoracic symmetry.

approach is used, the therapist will place both hands at the base of the chest with both thumbs pointing towards the xiphoid process of the sternum (Figure 44 and Figure 45). The clinician then asks the patient to take a deep breath and measures the distance from the thumb to the midline at the xiphoid process.

Using the posterior approach, the therapist will place the angle between the thumb and index finger at the inferior angle of the scapula with the thumbs pointing towards the spine

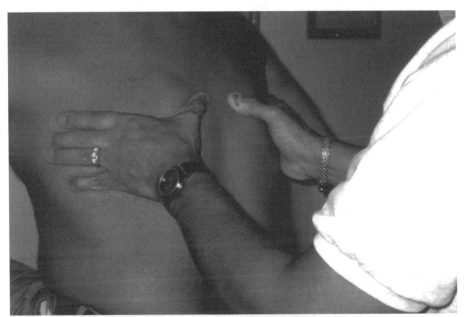

Figure 46: The posterior approach used to measure thoracic symmetry.

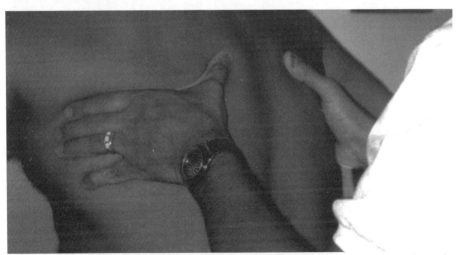

Figure 47: Close-up of the posterior approach used to measure thoracic symmetry.

(Figure 46 and Figure 47). The clinician performs the same test as in the anterior approach, measuring the bibasilar excursion of the thumbs from the midline, which in this case is represented by the spine.

A unilateral discrepancy in thoracic symmetry would suggest the possibility of decreased ventilatory capacity or atelectasis. Testing the strength of lateral basal chest excursions is simple and highly recommended at this point. It only requires applying some degree of resistance to the inspiratory effort of the patient using the techniques applied to measure bibasilar excursions for thoracic symmetry.

The strength of the intercostal muscles may be graded subjectively as good, fair, or poor. Diaphragmatic function should also be assessed by placing the ulnar border of one hand against the inferior border of the thorax and exerting moderate pressure in the direction of the diaphragmatic dome (Figure 48). The patient is asked to take a deep breath and the diaphragm is felt as it descends on inspiration. Strength can be determined with some degree of pressure or resistance and the same subjective grades can be used.

Functional Assessment

The Analysis of Gait

Gait analysis is a vital component of the overall functional evaluation. First, the ambulatory and weight-bearing status of the patient must be established. Then a critical analysis of the patient's gait pattern should be completed in the frontal and sagittal planes of progression (Figure 49). Displacements in the stance and swing phases

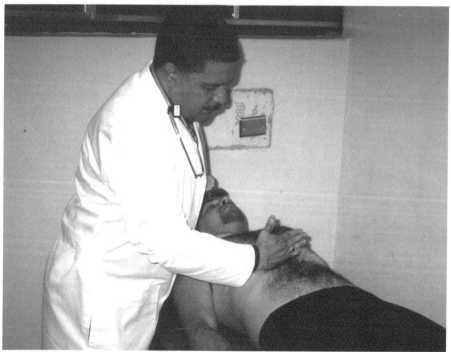

Figure 48: Assessing diaphragmatic function.

and subphases of gait are documented. This requires a kinetic analysis of the various muscle groups acting in these phases and comprehensive knowledge of the biomechanics of gait.

An evaluation of bed mobility and transfers would be particularly valuable for patients who are not ambulatory or for those who present with extremely high levels of pain. If the patient is not independent in these, the amount of assistance required to complete the activity should be documented.

In the process of completing a functional assessment, the therapist should inspect the patient's body mechanics in the various activities to identify bad habits in lifting, carrying, and in lying down. This is especially helpful for worker's compensation cases referred with low back or spinal injuries.

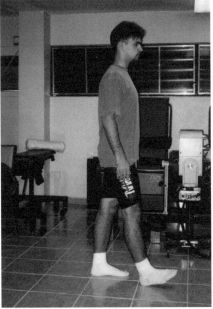

Figure 49: Analyzing gait in the sagittal plane of progression.

Selection of Functional Goals and Plan of Care Interventions

Once all the components of the DASI Pre-Aquatic Assessment have been completed, the relevant tests have been performed, and the clinical problems identified, the next step in the evaluation process is the establishment of goals. The Diagnostic Aquatics Systems Integration approach is concerned with a specific identification of a functional problem for which an intervention will be selected to address the dysfunction. Even though the DASI evaluation form focuses on the implementation of basic protocols and advanced aquatic rehabilitation interventions, it lists selected "land therapy" modalities and procedures that are integrated as a supplement to the aquatic therapy plan of care. The objective of these is to enhance the resolution of the clinical problem or problems.

Post-Aquatic Therapy Assessment

The Diagnostic Aquatic Systems Integration theory is concerned with the attainment of functional outcomes. Towards the end of the patient's referral period, another assessment should be completed; this time it will be called the Post-Aquatic Assessment (Appendix 2). This post-aquatic assessment addresses the same areas and integrates the same tests that were performed in the pre-aquatic phase. It is meant to provide accurate documentation concerning improvement in the identified functional deficits and clinical problems. However, the highlight of this document is the functional outcomes attainment where goals are once again listed and the therapist decides the percentage of improvement in each goal.

Based on the goals achieved and the extent of functional improvement, the therapist will decide the applicable recommendations, which will range from full discharge to determination of additional need for treatment.

Documentation in Aquatic Therapy

As in any other aspect of health care, documentation is of great importance in aquatic therapy. It provides the members of the health care team with a communication medium regarding the patient's progress and confirms the attainment of outcomes.

Considering the daily workload in the schedule of aquatic therapists, documentation can become a burdensome task. Consequently, problems in meeting deadlines for submission of progress notes and reports might occur. In order to minimize the occurrence of this situation, I have developed a concise form for daily documentation. The progress note model (Appendix 3) is described in the DASI approach to patient care. The format for documenting daily progress is similar to the format used for documentation in the initial and follow-up evaluations.

For patients with history of hypertension, pre- and post-activity blood pressure monitoring is strongly advised. DASI suggest the use of a flow sheet that is provided for that purpose (Appendix 4). This flow sheet can assist the therapist with clinical decision-making. For instance, if the pre-activity resting blood pressure reading is exceedingly high, considering the patient's baseline blood pressure, this will contraindicate treatment for that day and the patient will be placed on hold. Other land-based relaxation strategies might be utilized in an effort to lower the blood pressure before the decision to place the patient on hold is made.

Conclusion

The Diagnostic Aquatics Systems Integration Pre- and Post-Aquatic Assessments are two comprehensive instruments that emphasize identification of problems relevant not only to the patient's diagnosis but also to the identification of other underlying medical problems and past medical history. The secondary clinical problems that are identified in the evaluation will have an impact on goal establishment, treatment outcomes, and the design of the plan of care.

Section II

Aquatic Therapy Interventions

CHAPTER 3

BASIC AQUATIC THERAPY PROTOCOLS

Once the therapist has completed the initial pre-aquatic evaluation of the patient, the goals have been established, and the plan of care has been designed, the next step is to introduce the patient to basic activities in shallow water. In doing so, the patient will become familiar with and accustomed to the aquatic environment. This is considered an initial phase of adjustment for the patient.

The most common activities that are part of the initial protocol for patients consist of a variety of gait patterns and active stretching maneuvers. Gait patterns performed in shallow water have specific objectives and address specific clinical problems. Therefore, we must carefully select which gait patterns are beneficial for our patient because the wrong ambulatory pattern might be detrimental. For instance, patients with total hip arthroplasties should not practice any gait pattern that calls for adduction, internal

rotation beyond the midline, or excessive abduction with external rotation.

Basic activities can also be considered as warm-up exercises. In order to optimize soft tissue performance, active stretching of soft tissue structures is strongly advised before engaging in more dynamic activities. Lower extremity muscle groups are particularly important.

During the first aquatic therapy session, a great deal of emphasis should be placed on postural alignment with emphasis on the postural deficits identified in the pre-aquatic assessment.

Stretching Maneuvers

Passive and active stretching exercises in shallow water should be performed in three to four feet of water for optimal effectiveness. Equipment might help maximize the stretch but usually no equipment is needed. The stretch should be sustained for eight to ten

41

seconds. Depending on the extent of hamstring tightness, repetitions could vary from ten to twenty-five.

The Hamstrings Stretch

The most effective stretching maneuver for the hamstring muscles is a passive stretch achieved through the use of buoyant cuffs, which are fastened around the ankles, allowing the entire limb to float horizontally and at a right angle with the trunk. The patient should seek stabilization of the hip and trunk against the wall and let the extremity rise with the knee extended (Figure 50).

The Iliopsoas and Achilles Tendon Stretch

Tightening of the iliopsoas can be a source of excessive anterior hip rotation. However, one of the components of the quadriceps femoris muscle, the rectus femoris, can also exhibit tightening leading to anterior pelvic rotation. Stretching these soft tissue structures decreases postural deficits caused by tightening of its myofibrils. It is also important to stretch the connective tissue in order to maintain its plastic deformation properties. The function of the plantar flexors during heel strike, midstance, and push-off adds to the significance of their role during the gait cycle. When performing this stretch, the patient stands with one leg in hip hyperextension. The other leg is positioned in a forward step with the hip and knee flexed (Figure 51). Both feet should be flat on the bottom surface of the pool. With the hands holding onto the thigh on the flexed limb or the wall, the patient increases knee flexion thereby increasing the degree of extension on the opposite limb. Full contact of the plantar surfaces of both feet with the bottom surface of the pool should be maintained throughout the stretch.

The Tensor Fascia Latae and Gluteus Medius Stretch

While the iliopsoas is a deep flexor of the hip, the tensor fascia latae (TFL)

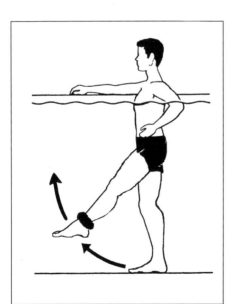

Figure 50: The hamstring stretch.

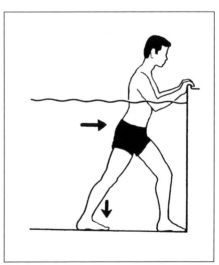

Figure 51: The iliopsoas and Achilles tendon stretch.

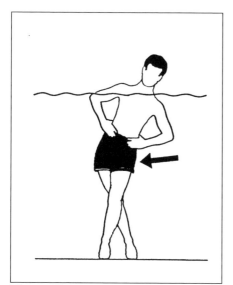

Figure 52: The tensor fascia latae and gluteus medius stretch.

is considered a superficial hip flexor along with the sartorius. The stretching technique for the TFL will also affect the gluteus medius muscle due to the position of the stretched leg. The patient stands with the leg to be stretched crossed over and behind the other leg. For upper body support, the patient may hold the edge of the pool deck or handrail. Assuming and maintaining this position will produce a static stretch of the TFL and gluteus medius. However, if we want to intensify the stretch, we can ask the patient to laterally flex the trunk to the opposite direction of the stretched TFL (Figure 52). Additionally, this stretching exercise will contribute to the release of a tight iliotibial band (IT band).

The Piriformis Stretch

As the primary external rotator of the hip, the piriformis muscle is the cause of clinical manifestations suggesting sciatic nerve pathology. The sciatic nerve courses directly under the piriformis muscle. Therefore, tightening or spasmodic activity of this muscle will cause undue compression of the sciatic nerve leading to the same clinical manifestations as sciatica secondary to a lumbar radiculopathy. Consequently, the piriformis stretch is one of the most important stretching maneuvers that must be considered in the warm-up program of aquatic activities. Collectively, the clinical manifestations caused by intense spasmodic activity of the piriformis (causing compression and impingement of the sciatic nerve and leading to localized and radiated pain, along with other related sensory-motor clinical signs) are referred to as the piriformis syndrome.

There are several ways to stretch the piriformis:

1. The patient can sit on the pool stair or on a pool bench. The extremity to be stretched is lifted and crossed so that the knee is flexed and the foot is resting on the opposite knee. With the opposite hand the patient pulls the flexed knee in an upward and inward direction towards the opposite pelvis (Figure 53 and Figure 54).
2. The patient stands and bends the hip and knee of the extremity to be stretched resting the foot on the opposite extended knee. Then, the patient is instructed to internally rotate the hip by moving the knee medially (Figure 55).

The Hip Adductor Stretch

Tightness of the proximal hip adductor group restricts range of motion and flexibility of the hip. This group consists of the pectineus, adductor magnus, adductor longus, adductor brevis, and gracilis. Of these, the pecti-

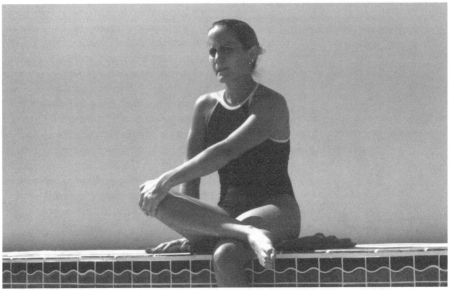

Figure 53: Sitting technique for the piriformis stretch, starting position.

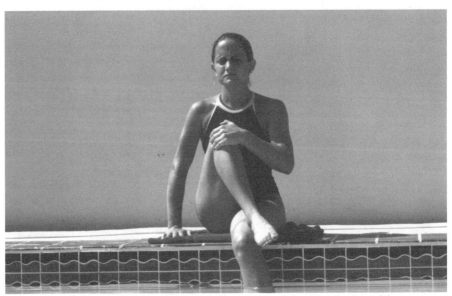

Figure 54: Sitting technique for the piriformis stretch, stretched position.

neus, the most proximally located of all, can be a particularly problematic soft tissue structure when it is spasmodic. It causes a characteristic burning pain along with limited range of motion, and decreased flexibility.

Two exercises are used to stretch the pectineus and other adductor muscles:

1. In shallow water, the patient stands with a considerably wide base of support and the extremity to be

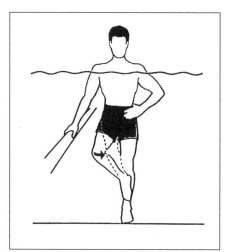

Figure 55: Standing technique for the piriformis stretch.

stretched extended. The feet are in full contact with the bottom surface of the pool. He is instructed to move the body towards the opposite side while flexing the knee (Figure 56). This maneuver stretches all the adductor muscles.

2. In deep water, the patient must wear a floatation belt to allow vertical floatation and suspension.

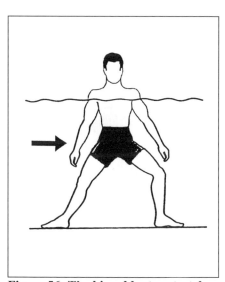

Figure 56: The hip adductor stretch.

This stretch is most effective if practiced in six to ten feet of water. The patient is instructed to bring both heels together with the plantar surfaces of the feet touching each other. This position will result in external rotation of both hips and knee flexion. The patient moves the heels up towards the pelvis increasing knee flexion, hip abduction, and external rotation (Figure 57). This maneuver is especially effective for pectineus tightness and is referred to as the groin stretch.

Shallow-Water Dynamic Gait Activities

Depending on the gait patterns selected by the aquatic therapist and the prescribed laps, shallow-water dynamic gait activities might last between 15 and 30 minutes. Patients with low back pain or sciatica might experience an increase in pain level with decreased tolerance to certain types of aquatic gait patterns. The therapist must exercise

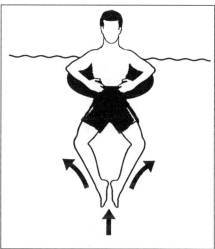

Figure 57: The deep-water groin stretch or pectineus stretch.

careful judgment when deciding which type of gait pattern is indicated or contraindicated for the patient. Gait activities can be modified. For instance, seated gait activities in shallow water using the floatation noodle or deep-water jogging activities are a suitable substitute if the patient has reported an increase in pain levels while practicing an aquatic gait pattern. The impact on the lumbar spine and pelvis is significantly decreased and the exercises improve the rhythm and the lumbar-pelvic alignment.

Resisted forward and retrogait activities are advised if the goal is to increase cardiovascular endurance, improve trunk stability and motor control, improve dynamic balance, and increase strength. A wide selection of resistive aquatic equipment such as paddles, dumbbells, and boards will make the activity more challenging.

Forward Gait

When a patient is walking forward in shallow water, we must emphasize posture and pattern. There are two rules to follow. First, encourage the patient to walk with a reference upright posture. The shoulders should be aligned with the hips. When we ambulate, there is a certain amount of arm swing. Therefore, in the water we should replicate our gait pattern on land by coordinating leg and arm movements; that is, we should follow a pattern reflecting synchronous movement of the right upper extremity with the left lower extremity.

Second, encourage awareness of the walking pattern, pointing out that in the water the patient will be ambulating in "slow motion" as compared to ambulating on land. Follow the heel strike to push-off sequence, that is, heel to toe with the metatarsal break (Figure 58).

Retrogait

This activity reverses the sequence to a toe to heel backward direction. Begin at toe off (push off) and proceed

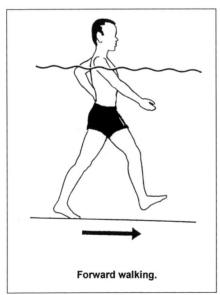

Forward walking.

Figure 58: Forward gait in shallow water.

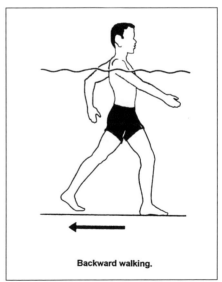

Backward walking.

Figure 59: Retrogait in shallow water.

to midstance and heel touch. Arm coordination continues to follow lower extremity movement. When the right leg moves backward so does the left arm (Figure 59).

If the patient is experiencing severe localized or radiated pain rendering him unable to performing these types of weight-bearing activities, apply floatation equipment and proceed with deep-water dynamic activities.

Side-Stepping Gait

The patient is standing with a six to ten inch base of support. The toes and hips are facing forward. Instruct the patient to take a side step abducting one lower extremity and widening the base of support (Figure 60). The arms should be abducted slightly as the patient abducts the lower limb to take the side step. Then, the opposite leg and arm are adducted toward the leg that initiated the side step. At this point, the legs

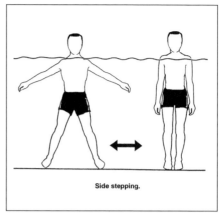

Side stepping.

Figure 60: The side-stepping gait.

should be only shoulder width apart. Be careful not to allow excessive rotation of the pelvis on a transverse plane.

The therapist should observe the position of each foot as the patient takes the side step. If the feet are not properly aligned, this has a negative influence on the patient's posture and will impact the level of pain. This is an important

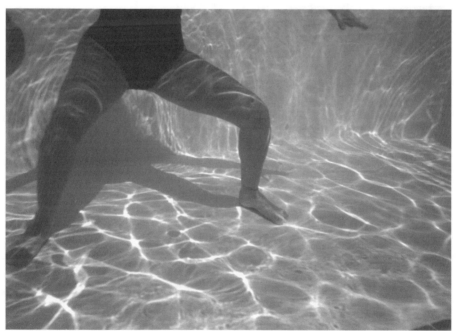

Figure 61: The side-stepping crab walk.

consideration in patients with low back pain.

A variation of this side-stepping gait pattern, which is characterized by marked flexion of the knees and hips with each side step, is known as the crab walk (Figure 61). If the patient experiences difficulty or discomfort when performing a crab walk, a flotation noodle can be used. The patient sits on the flotation noodle and proceeds with a side-stepping crab walk. Other types of crabwalk include the forward and retro crab walk (Figure 62). To promote pelvic and trunk control, the degree of difficulty can be increased with use of resistive aquatic equipment such as boards, paddles, or dumbbells.

The aquatic therapist should decide which type of side-stepping gait pattern is more appropriate for the patient depending on the patient's history and the clinical problems identified on the patient's pre-aquatic assessment.

The High Knee or Marching Gait

This type of forward aquatic gait pattern resembles a forward march. One hip and knee are flexed as the patient moves forward in combination with

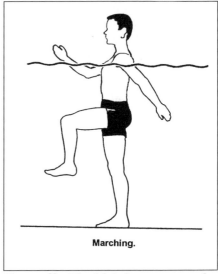

Marching.

Figure 63: The high knee or marching gait.

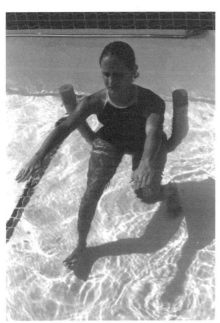

Figure 62: The seated noodle crab walk (forward and retro).

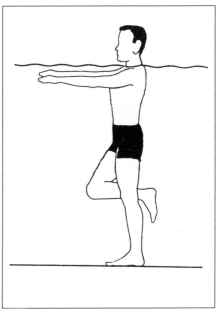

Figure 64: The stork stand.

modified forward breaststrokes at water surface level (Figure 63). In order to promote coordination and correct posture in this type of gait pattern, the "stork stand" static posture exercise (Figure 64) should be practiced prior to instructing the patient on the marching movements.

Midline Gait

The patient abducts one leg while weight bearing on the other, simultaneously abducting both upper extremities. As he adducts that same leg to the midline of the body, he steps directly in front of the weight-bearing foot (Figure 65). The same sequence of movements is repeated on the opposite leg. This type of gait pattern challenges balance and trunk stability.

The tightrope gait is a variation of this type of aquatic gait pattern. In the tightrope gait, both shoulders are maintained in abduction to 90°.

Crossover Stepping or Braiding Gait

This type of aquatic gait is similar to the side-stepping pattern. However, the difference lies in that during adduction of the lower extremity, the patient crosses that leg over the weight-bearing limb, thereby crossing the midline (Figure 66).

Other Shallow-Water-Specific Exercises

The aquatic therapist should be creative in applying and designing activities and exercises for the patient based on the diagnosis, history, and clinical findings in the pre-aquatic assessment. The knowledge and expertise of the professional will allow him to exercise the appropriate clinical judgment given the circumstances.

For patients experiencing low back pain secondary to lumbar radiculopathy or herniation, application of land exercises might be a helpful predecessor to

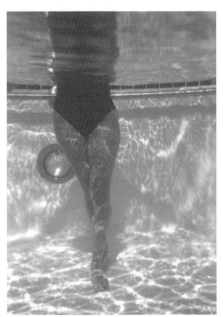

Figure 65: The midline gait.

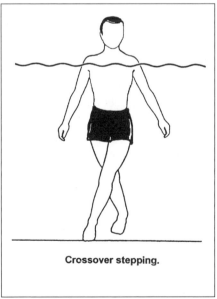

Crossover stepping.

Figure 66: The crossover stepping or braiding gait.

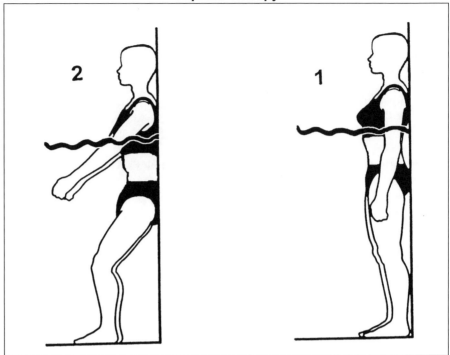

Figure 67: Pelvic tilt with wall slide.

other activities in shallow water. These applications include pelvic tilt exercises in the upright standing position or the wall slide exercise. The patient's back is against the wall as he performs a pelvic tilt and slides his back down to a 90° hip flexion position (Figure 67). Thereafter, he returns to the original position and releases the pelvic tilt.

Seated Noodle Exercises

Besides the crabwalk, seated noodle activities include pelvic tilt exercises in the sitting position, lateral pelvic shift in the sitting position (Figure 68), and "figure of eight" exercises in the sitting position. If the patient experiences difficulty performing a pelvic tilt in the upright position, it might be easier for the patient to do this activity while seated on the floatation noodle.

When performing seated noodle figure of eight exercises, the knees or buttocks are used as points of reference. The patient may hold the handrails while completing seated noodle exercises.

Deep-Water Dynamic Activities

If the patient is apprehensive of the water, it will take longer for him to adjust to the aquatic environment and be ready for deep-water activities. The patient will be ready when he is able to perform all of the shallow-water dynamic activities independently. The adjustment phase will vary in duration. When the patient begins deep-water activities, the entire first session and a number of subsequent sessions will center on adjustment to deep water.

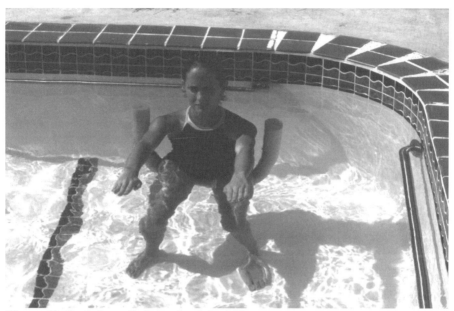

Figure 68: Seated noodle lateral pelvic shift.

For patients with reported high pain levels who demonstrate apprehension to the water, instead of beginning a program of deep-water activities, it is recommended to position the patient in the supine position with floatation equipment (belt, cervical collar, and ankle rings). In this position, a floatation noodle can be placed under the knees, promoting knee and hip flexion. This is one of the Bad Ragaz positions known as passive relaxation. Another effective technique consists of cradling the patient in preparation for selected Watsu® basic flow movement sequences.

For deep-water activities, the patient must wear a floatation pelvic belt or an AquaJogger. The belt must be properly aligned in order to provide optimal buoyancy and vertical suspension (Figure 69). The inferior border of the belt must rest upon the iliac crests. The center of the back of the belt must be in line with the sacrum. If the belt slides towards the chest it could restrict

the patient's breathing pattern. The belt buckles should be tightened so that the belt is kept in place. Do not tighten the

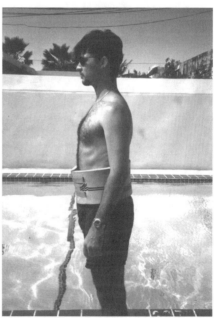

Figure 69: Correct application of floatation pelvic belt.

belt excessively as this could cause discomfort to the patient.

Deep-Water Jogging

Take the patient to the borderline of the shallow end that defines the beginning of the deep-water area. In deep water, buoyancy increases. Therefore, it will be more difficult for the patient to maintain postural alignment in the vertical upright position. The degree of difficulty will increase if the patient is obese, if the patient is an amputee, or if the patient has a neurological problem with flaccidity, spasticity, hemiplegia, or monoplegia.

Training the patient to align his body vertically in deep water begins with the "T" position (Figure 70). This position follows the pathway of the line of gravity. At this time, the therapist should inspect the postural alignment. The shoulders are at 90° abduction with

the lower extremities closely adducted and well aligned with the trunk. Try to maintain the body in vertical alignment.

Chin and head control is the key to maintaining a balanced vertical position in deep water. When possible, these applied recovery techniques should be used to train the patient to return to the upright vertical position if he has a tendency to roll backward or forward. If the patient has a tendency to roll on his back from the vertical position, recovery can be accomplished by bringing the chin towards the sternum. This is followed by hip and knee extension until a vertically aligned posture is assumed. If the patient's body rolls prone, cervical extension will bring about a vertically aligned position.

During deep-water jogging, the hands and the feet are the means of forward propulsion. Instruct the patient

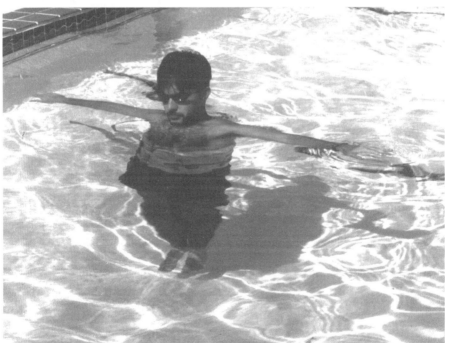

Figure 70: Deep-water vertical alignment in the "T" position.

to shape the hands in cylinder prehension as if he were holding a glass of water with the fingers close together (Figure 71). The wrists are kept in neutral position. Begin with the shoulders at 90° flexion. The arms are kept close to the trunk. The movement of the upper extremities consists of shoulder hyperextension with elbow flexion alternated with shoulder flexion and elbow extension of the opposite arm. The lower extremity movement sequence consists of hip and knee flexion with ankle dorsiflexion alternated in the opposite limb with hip and knee extension with ankle plantar flexion (Figure 72). The flexion sequence of the right lower extremity occurs simultaneously with the extension sequence of the left upper extremity and vice versa. If at all possible, practice the position of the upper and lower extremities and movements required for forward pro-pulsion in the shallow area.

The aquatic therapist must stay close to the patient while training the patient about deep-water dynamics until the patient can perform these activities correctly and independently. During the initial training in deep-water activities, the therapist should maintain contact guarding with the patient at least during the first series of laps and then gradually wean the patient towards independence. Verbal and manual cueing is an important strategy in this training.

Because of the weightlessness caused by buoyancy, the patient is predisposed to articular instability. If movements are performed incorrectly or body segments are incorrectly aligned, this could lead to an increase in pain levels and decreased tolerance of the activity. In deep water at shoulder level, the individual loses approximately ninety percent of his weight. Additionally, there is more cardiovas-

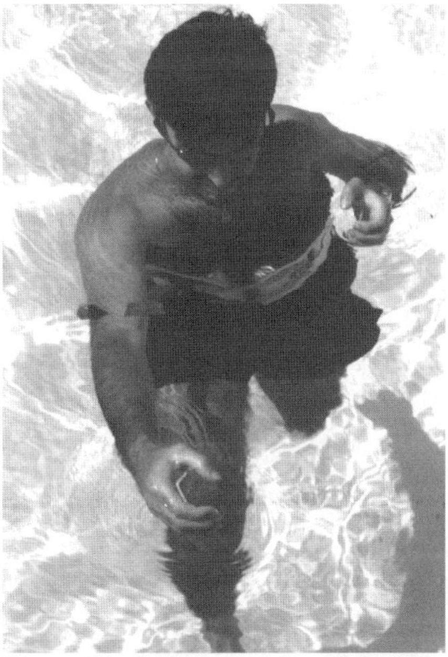

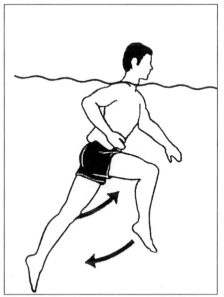

Figure 71: Cylinder prehension of the hand for deep-water forward propulsion.

Figure 72: Alternate and simultaneous movements of the upper and lower extremities in deep-water jogging.

cular effort required with increased demands for cardiac output. These two factors should be taken into consideration when preparing the patient for deep-water activities.

When proficiency in this activity is attained, laps may be completed at the discretion of the therapist. It is a common practice to instruct the patient to deep-water jog for a period of thirty minutes to an hour depending on the patient's condition and tolerance. However, it is extremely important for the patient to take frequent rest intervals between laps, as this will avoid early soft tissue and cardiopulmonary fatigue. Other clinical objectives that are related to forward deep-water jogging might involve improvement of motor control or strengthening of weak musculature. In order to address these goals later in the program, the therapist might consider adding resistance, either manual or with the aid of aquatic

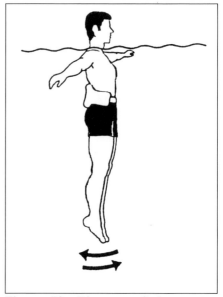

Figure 73: Diagram of deep-water vertical retroactivity with flutter kicks.

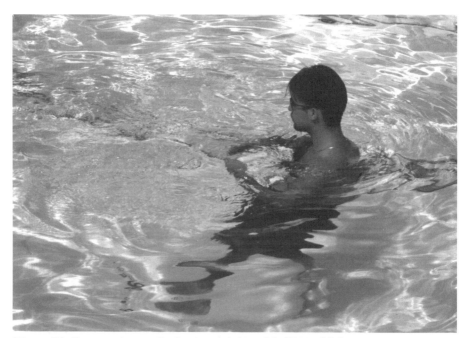

Figure 74: Deep-water vertical retroactivity with flutter kicks.

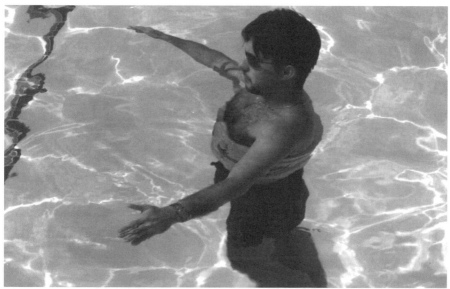

Figure 75: Upper extremity movements during deep-water vertical retroactivity, position 1.

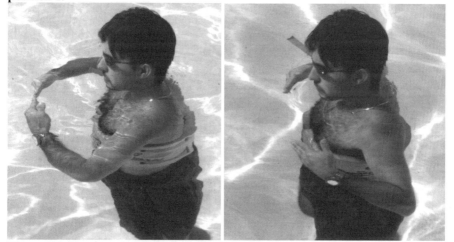

Figure 76: Upper extremity movements during deep-water vertical retroactivity, position 2 and position 3.

equipment to challenge motor control and strengthen weak muscles.

Deep-Water Vertical Retroactivity

The integration of retroactivity within deep-water dynamics is important in order to strengthen the extensors of the spine responsible for maintaining trunk stability. All types of patients, particularly those suffering from low back pain, need to practice retroactivity. Besides strengthening the erector spinae, vertical retroactivity in deep water is also effective in strengthening the anterolateral abdominal muscles. These muscle groups will co-contract synergistically to enhance balance and stability. In contrast to this, land-based exercises focus on strengthening the abdominals in comparison to the back muscles.

However, we must consider that the patient might not initially tolerate this activity if pain levels are high or the condition is acute. In that case, concentrate only on deep-water jogging in forward propulsion until the patient's condition allows integration of retroactivity. Some patients with radiculopathy, degenerative disc disease, or herniation might report an increase in pain and discomfort when performing retroactivity in deep water. If this technique continues to cause pain and discomfort, it should be removed from the aquatic plan of care and other, less strenuous activities that will achieve the same outcome in shallow or deep water should be substituted.

When the patient reaches the far edge of the pool deck after finishing a forward propulsion deep-water jog, instruct the patient to assume the "T" position once again with the toes pointing to the bottom of the pool and the knees extended (Figure 73 and Figure 74). A slight pelvic tilt should be performed to bring the body into a neutral alignment. The lower extremity movement will be a straight leg flutter kick. These flutter kicks involve activity of the superficial hip flexors with slight activity of the iliopsoas. The gluteus maximus is the most active antagonist in hip hyperextension during a flutter kick. The upper extremity movement is called the "squid arm"

activity. Practice of this movement should precede the flutter kicks. With both shoulders abducted at 90° and the elbows extended, instruct the patient to horizontally adduct the arms towards the midline forming two intertwining circles (Figure 75 and Figure 76). As the patient returns to the original position, the movement is repeated.

Avoid excessive shoulder horizontal abduction when returning to the original position. This will hyperextend the lumbar spine and place the pectoral muscles in an unsafe stretched position causing cervical and shoulder pain. Compensatory movements such as thoracic and cervical spine hyperextension or bilateral shoulder and scapular elevation should also be avoided because these will render the activity ineffective. The "squid arm" activities in combination with the flutter kicks are the primary means of backward propulsion for deep-water vertical retroactivity.

Conclusion

Basic aquatic therapy activities provide the basis for patient adjustment to the aquatic environment and serve as preparatory protocols for other aquatic therapy interventions.

Shallow-water dynamic activities focus on gait and specific exercises while deep-water dynamic activities require more stability and control to maintain a vertically aligned balance.

CHAPTER 4

BAD RAGAZ RING METHOD

History and Perspective

In the 1930s, a program of aquatic exercises was implemented in the town of Bad Ragaz, Switzerland. Later, in 1957, a German doctor revised and developed the Bad Ragaz protocol. He added a stabilization component provided by three floatation rings at the neck, pelvis, and ankles. He developed and integrated structured patterns that consisted of passive, active, active assistive, and resistive movements. These patterns evolved into what is known today as the Bad Ragaz Ring Method.

Bad Ragaz Patterns

Bad Ragaz patterns integrate proprioceptive neuromuscular facilitation concepts. Each pattern can be modified and adapted to a large variety of orthopedic or neurological diagnoses. While still implementing some of the original concepts, the most commonly used Bad Ragaz patterns allow better control and hand placement for the aquatic therapist, enhancing the ability to facilitate or inhibit a response. There is a large selection of patterns based on the patient's clinical problems and pre-established functional goals. The patterns featured in the Bad Ragaz Ring Method are grouped in three categories: lower extremity, trunk, and upper extremity.

Another classification divides the applied techniques into passive and command patterns. Passive patterns do not require any active participation by the patient. Command patterns require the patient to have intact cognitive abilities in order to be perform the patterns adequately. If the ability to comprehend a command has been altered (e.g., patients with receptive aphasia), the patient will not be able to perform any of these patterns. When a command pattern is used, the therapist instructs the patient to perform a specific movement. If the patient is unable to perform the movement upon command, the pattern will not be effective.

A considerable list of Bad Ragaz patterns have been identified. The twenty patterns described in this chapter are the ones I consider to be the most commonly used in aquatic rehabilitation.

Objectives and Precautions

When the objective is focused on neuromuscular re-education, the applied principle of the stretch reflex can be integrated to improve contractile properties and strength in a single muscle or in muscle groups.

Even though the Diagnostic Aquatics Systems Integration approach does not contraindicate the application of Bad Ragaz in upper motor neuron

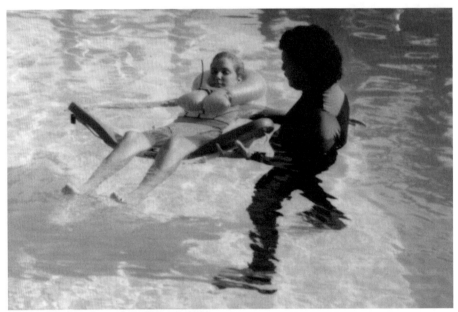

Figure 77: Passive relaxation position.

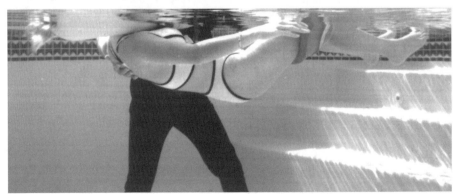

Figure 78: Underwater view of the passive relaxation position.

disorders, it is strongly advised to carefully select and apply these patterns. In neurological cases, some patterns might increase hypertonicity. Furthermore, the application of Bad Ragaz patterns in a patient with loss of function due to a stroke is not contraindicated. On the contrary, it could prove very beneficial in the neuromuscular re-education of the hemiplegic or hemiparetic limbs. Caution should be exercised when trunk patterns are applied, particularly in patients with spinal surgery.

Application Guidelines

The recommended water depth for efficient and effective application of Bad Ragaz is three to four feet. The water level should remain within the therapist's T8 to T11 vertebrae. A rise in water level above T8 would result in a loss of stability for the therapist. The clinician would have to work harder against the effects of buoyancy.

The Diagnostic Aquatics Systems Integration approach utilizes a selected number of described upper extremity, lower extremity, and trunk patterns based on successful outcomes in a variety of patients with orthopedic and neurological conditions. Some are command and others are passive. These patterns are categorically and descriptively presented below.

Passive Relaxation

DASI advocates the use of the passive relaxation position (Figure 77 and Figure 78) on patients with radiculopathy experiencing a high level of low back pain or as a treatment closure technique. This is not a pattern but a specific position aimed at promoting relaxation and relieving pain. The patient is in the supine position. A cervical floatation collar and a pelvic floatation belt are worn. A floatation noodle is placed under the patient's knees to maintain a certain degree of knee and hip flexion, thereby releasing the pressure in the lumbar spine. The passive relaxation position could also benefit patients with lower extremity extensor spasticity.

The pelvic and trunk patterns are shown, starting on the next page. On the following pages are the lower extremity patterns and the upper extremity patterns.

Pelvic and Trunk Patterns

Passive Pelvic Tilt

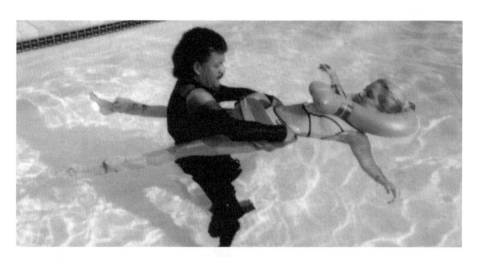

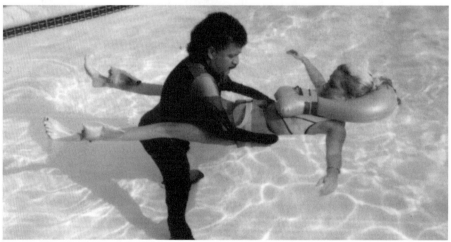

Figure 79: Passive pelvic tilt.

Position of Patient	Supine wearing floatation collar, pelvic belt, and ankle rings.
Position of Therapist	Standing between the patient's thighs.
Hand Placement	Thumbs at anterior superior iliac spine (ASIS) with the four medial digits around the iliac crest.
Technique	Push down on ASIS tilting the pelvis posteriorly. Allow the pelvis to return to its original anterior tilt.

Passive Trunk Elongation with Pelvic Hold

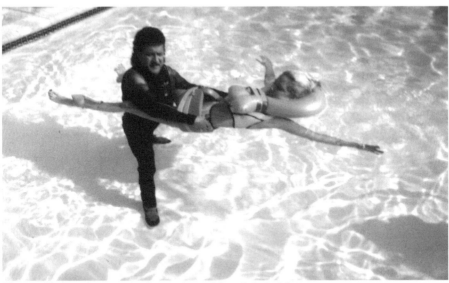

Figure 80: Passive trunk elongation with pelvic hold.

Position of Patient	Supine wearing floatation collar, pelvic belt, and ankle rings.
Position of Therapist	Standing between the patient's thighs. The therapist should maintain a wide base of support.
Hand Placement	Around iliac crests.
Technique	Rock the patient from side to side. Allow approximately 180° of lateral movement of the trunk on the water. Pull caudally on each iliac crest alternately for facilitation of the lateral trunk muscles. To facilitate unilateral trunk rotation, push one innominate bone posteriorly at the ASIS while pushing on the PSIS (posterior superior iliac spine) of the opposite os coxae.

Passive Trunk Elongation with Knee Hold

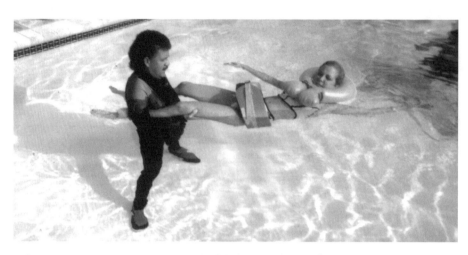

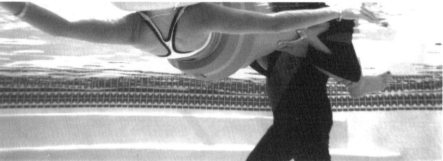

Figure 81: Passive trunk elongation with knee hold.

Position of Patient	Supine wearing floatation collar, pelvic belt, and ankle rings.
Position of Therapist	Standing between the patient's legs below the knees. The therapist should maintain a wide base of support.
Hand Placement	Posterolaterally at the popliteal fossa. Maintain slight hip and knee flexion with external rotation.
Technique	Rock the patient from side to side. Allow approximately 180° of lateral movement of the trunk on the water. Unilaterally pull down on knee in the caudal direction on the posterior aspect of the tibial condyles causing distraction of the articular surfaces of the knee joint while performing approximation of the opposite knee joint surfaces. Observe the movement of the lateral trunk, hip, and thigh on the water.

Passive Trunk Elongation with Thoracic Hold

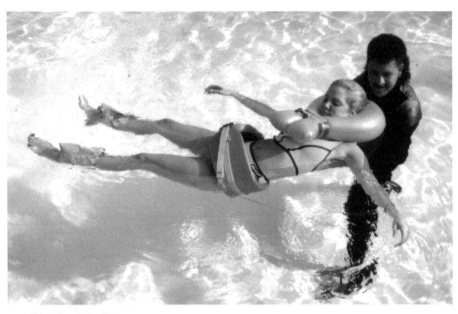

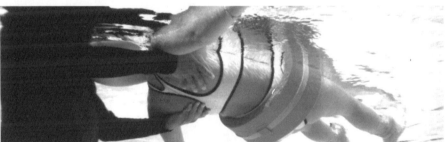

Figure 82: Passive trunk elongation with thoracic hold

Position of Patient	Supine wearing floatation collar, pelvic belt, and ankle rings.
Position of Therapist	Standing at the head of the patient. The therapist should maintain a wide base of support.
Hand Placement	Posterior thorax and scapular region with thumbs near the axillary fold.
Technique	Move the patient gently from side to side through the water covering approximately 180°. Observe the stretch of the lateral trunk and hip muscles. Gentle rotation can be added to this pattern by pushing down on one side and up on the opposite side, then alternating the movement.

Passive Trunk Elongation with Elbow Hold

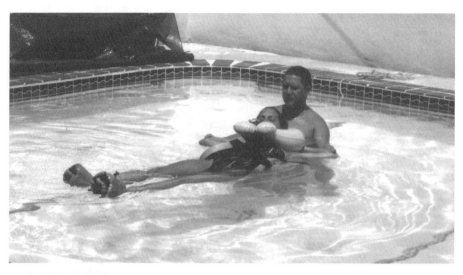

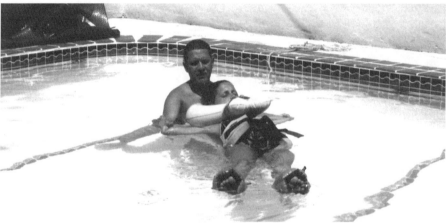

Figure 83: Passive trunk elongation with elbow hold.

Position of Patient	Supine wearing floatation collar, pelvic belt, and ankle rings. Both hands are grasping the floatation collar with elbows in full flexion, shoulders externally rotated.
Position of Therapist	Standing at the head of the patient. The therapist should maintain a wide base of support.
Hand Placement	At the patient's elbows.
Technique	Gently move the patient from side to side covering approximately 180° of surface area. Observe the stretch in the scapular and lateral trunk muscles.

Isotonic #1

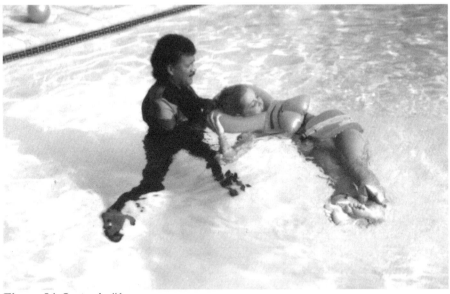

Figure 84: Isotonic #1.

Position of Patient	Supine wearing floatation collar, pelvic belt, and ankle rings. Hands at the sides holding the floatation collar with elbows flexed.
Position of Therapist	Standing at the patient's head. The therapist should maintain a wide base of support.
Hand Placement	At the patient's elbows.
Command	"Keep your knees straight. Point your toes up towards the ceiling. Drop your right hip and bring your legs and toes toward your right elbow." Repeat the same command on the left side.
Technique	Move the patient to the right to decrease resistance or to the left to increase resistance. Repeat the technique on the left side.

Isotonic #2

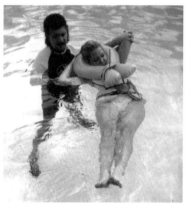
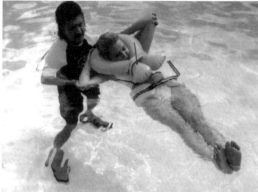
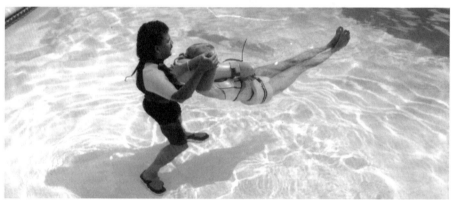

Figure 85: Isotonic #2.

Position of Patient	Supine wearing floatation collar, pelvic belt, and ankle rings. Hands over the head and holding the floatation collar with elbows flexed.
Position of Therapist	Standing at the patient's head.
Hand Placement	At the patient's elbows.
Command	"Keep your knees straight. Point your toes up towards the ceiling. Bring your hips up. Now keeping your legs close together bring them towards the left." Repeat to the right.
Technique	Stabilize the patient at the elbows and follow the direction of the patient's movement through the water to decrease resistance. Moving in the opposite direction will increase resistance.

Isometric

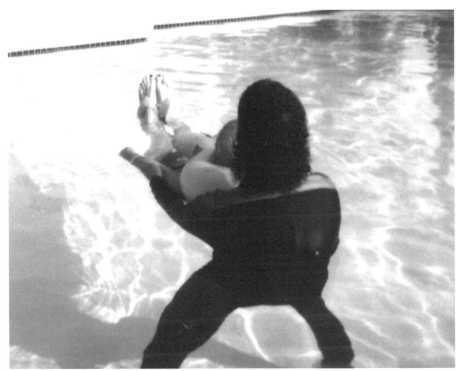

Figure 86: Isometric.

Position of Patient	Supine wearing floatation collar, pelvic belt, and ankle rings. Arms at the sides of the body with extended elbows.
Position of Therapist	Standing at the patient's head.
Hand Placement	At the posterior thorax and scapular regions with thumbs near the axillary fold.
Command	"Keep your knees straight. Point your toes up towards the ceiling. Bring your hips up and hold that position while I move you through the water. Hold…hold…relax."
Technique	Move the patient to the left and then to the right gradually increasing speed and resistance.

Lower Extremity Patterns

Tone Inhibition

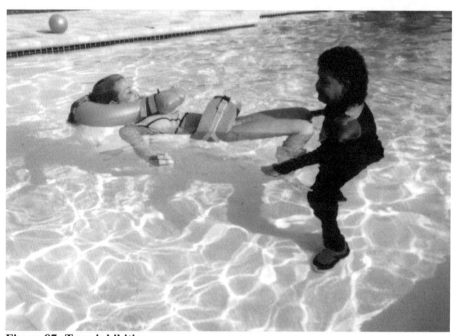

Figure 87: Tone inhibition.

Position of Patient	Supine wearing floatation collar, pelvic belt, and ankle rings. Hips and knees must be extended.
Position of Therapist	Standing at the feet of the patient.
Hand Placement	At first in the extension position, hands are at the dorsum of feet. During the pattern movements, the hands move to the heels of the feet.
Technique	The therapist moves forward towards the patient and squats into the cube position, allowing the patient's feet to drop with bilateral knee flexion and hip external rotation. This pattern is generally applied as a passive pattern but it can become a command pattern if the patient can voluntarily recruit motor activity. In that case, the command would be, "Keep your hip up. Bend your knees and drop your heels down and back."

Pre-Weight-Bearing

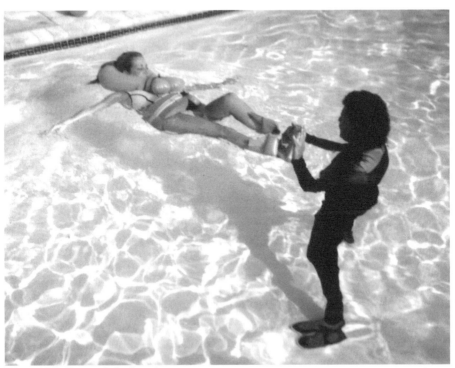

Figure 88: Pre-weight-bearing.

Position of Patient	Supine wearing floatation collar, pelvic belt, and ankle rings.
Position of Therapist	Standing at the patient's feet.
Hand Placement	One hand is holding on the dorsum of one foot while the plantar surface of the opposite foot is resting on therapist's other hand.
Command	"Push the foot that is resting on my hand down toward me keeping the knee straight. Now at the same time pull your other foot up towards you while you bend the knee, pulling my hand up with your foot. Hold...hold...hold...relax."
Technique	On the extended leg resist plantar flexion while simultaneously resisting dorsiflexion on the opposite foot.

Pre-Gait

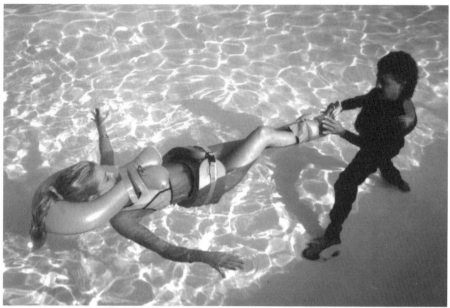

Figure 89: Pre-gait.

Position of Patient	Supine wearing floatation collar, pelvic belt, and ankle rings.
Position of Therapist	Standing at the patient's feet.
Hand Placement	Fingers at dorsum of the patient's feet with thumbs at the plantar surface of the metatarsal heads.
Command	"Push on my thumb with the ball of your right foot keeping your knee straight. At the same time pull your left foot up towards you bringing my fingers up and slightly bending your hip and knee. Now pull your right foot up and your left foot down…now switch again…up and down…and switch again…relax."
Technique	The therapist resists ankle dorsiflexion on the left foot while simultaneously resisting ankle plantar flexion on the right foot. As the patient becomes proficient in performing the alternate ankle motions, he may be instructed to integrate alternate slight knee and hip flexion with extension. The therapist might consider walking towards the patient as the movements are performed.

Unilateral Lower Extremity

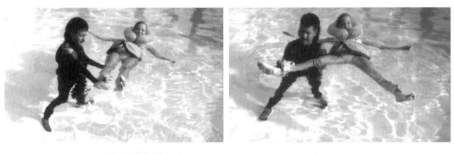

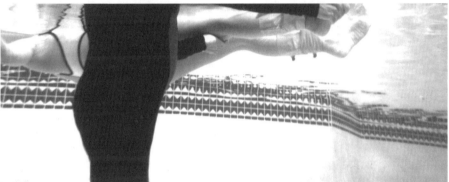

Figure 90: Unilateral lower extremity.

Position of Patient	Supine wearing floatation collar, pelvic belt, and ankle rings. The hip on the affected leg is extended, adducted, and internally rotated with the knee extended.
Position of Therapist	Standing facing the affected leg.
Hand Placement	The proximal hand is on the lateral surface of the distal thigh and the distal hand is on the lateral aspect of the foot.
Command	"With your toes pointing up, turn your foot out and push your entire leg out and away from the other one against my hands. Now switch and bring your leg in towards the other one turning your foot in."
Technique	The therapist acts as a stabilizer, guiding the lower extremity into hip extension, abduction, and external rotation with the knee extended and the foot everted against resistance or without resistance. Hand placement is then moved to the medial aspect of the thigh and foot while the patient adducts and internally rotates the leg with foot inversion.

Bilateral Lower Extremity

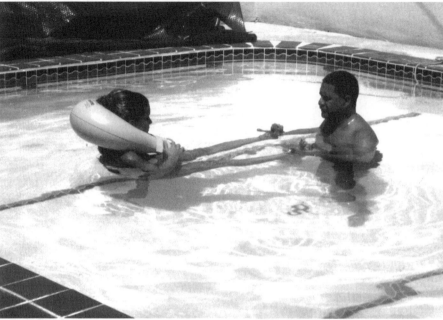

Figure 91: Bilateral lower extremity.

Position of Patient	Supine wearing floatation collar, pelvic belt, and ankle rings. The hips are extended, adducted, and internally rotated with the knee extended.
Position of Therapist	Standing at the feet of the patient.
Hand Placement	On the medial aspect of both feet.
Command	"Turn your foot out and push both legs out and away against my hands. At the same time, bring your trunk up to a long sitting position. Hold…hold…hold…and relax."
Technique	The therapist switches his hand placement to the lateral aspect of both feet in order to resist hip abduction, external rotation, and foot eversion. This pattern can be performed without resistance if the emphasis is on the re-education of the abdominal muscles. The patient is allowed to hold the floatation collar while performing trunk flexion.

Bilateral Symmetrical Lower Extremity #1

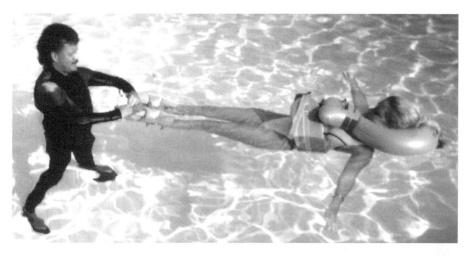

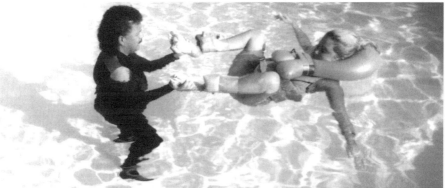

Figure 92: Bilateral symmetrical lower extremity #1.

Position of Patient	Supine wearing floatation collar, pelvic belt, and ankle rings. Both hips are in extension and internal rotation with knee extension, ankle plantar flexion, and inversion.
Position of Therapist	Standing at the patient's feet.
Hand Placement	Both hands on the dorsum of the patient's feet with the fingers pointing to the medial border and the thenar and hypothenar eminences pointing to the lateral border.
Command	"Pull your toes up and out. At the same time, bend your knees up and out. Lift your head, neck, and chest and bring it towards your knees."
Technique	The patient moves the trunk into flexion with simultaneous knee flexion, hip flexion, hip abduction and external rotation, ankle dorsiflexion and eversion. This pattern can be applied without considering its sequel (#2).

Bilateral Symmetrical Lower Extremity #2

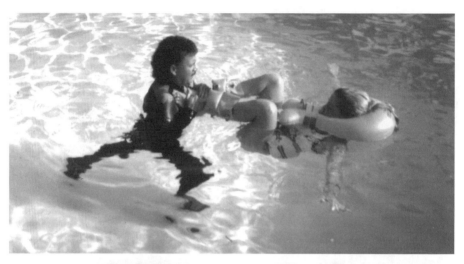

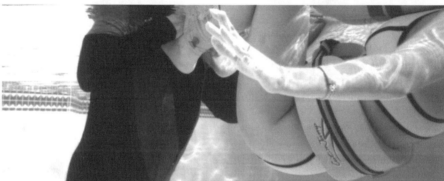

Figure 93: Bilateral symmetrical lower extremity #2

Position of Patient	Supine wearing floatation collar, pelvic belt, and ankle rings. Both hips are flexed, abducted, and externally rotated with the trunk and knees flexed.
Position of Therapist	Standing at the patient's feet.
Hand Placement	Dorsum of both feet with feet resting either on one of the therapist's hips or on the therapist upper chest.
Command	"Push your head and trunk back while at the same time pushing your toes/feet against my chest/hip."
Technique	The patient moves the head back into the supine position extending the spine, hips, and knees with hip adduction and internal rotation. These movements are performed against the resistance offered by the therapist's hip/chest. This pattern is the continuation of the bilateral symmetrical lower extremity #1 pattern.

Bilateral Reciprocal Lower Extremity

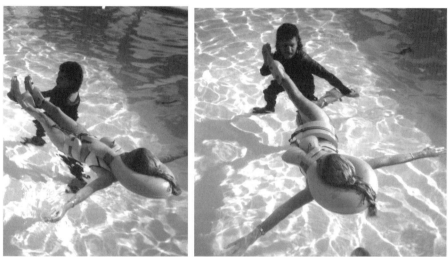

Figure 94: Bilateral reciprocal lower extremity.

Position of Patient	Supine wearing floatation collar, pelvic belt, and ankle rings with both lower extremities in hip extension, adduction, and knee extension.
Position of Therapist	Standing at the patient's feet facing the patient's right foot.
Hand Placement	The right hand on placed on the sole of the patient's right foot. The left hand is holding the left heel.
Command	"Bring your right toes up. Then, push your left heel against my hand while you drop your hip, bringing your left foot down and under your right leg to the other side."
Technique	The therapist performs approximation of knee joint surfaces on the right leg while guiding the left heel into the water and under the right leg. The patient can also be allowed to actively perform the command without guidance from the therapist. Resistance can also be added for strengthening purposes. The pattern allows unilateral re-education and/or strengthening of an affected lower extremity. If the emphasis is on bilateral re-education, a switch in hand placement is necessary.

Upper Extremity Patterns

Unilateral Upper Extremity

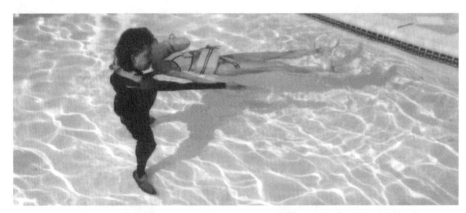

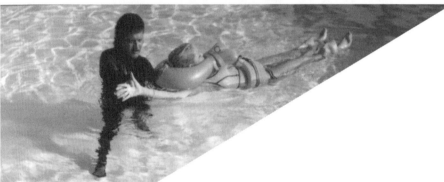

Figure 95: Unilateral upper extremity.

Position of Patient	Supine wearing floatation collar, pelvic belt, and ankle rings. Both arms must be in shoulder extension, adduction, and internal rotation with forearm pronation and finger flexion.
Position of Therapist	Standing at the patient's right side.
Hand Placement	The therapist's left hand is supporting the patient's scapula while the right hand is either over the patient's fingers of the fisted right hand or holding the patient's right hand at his palm.
Command	"Keep your elbow straight. Open your fingers. Turn your palm up and push your hand and arm out and back against my hand."
Technique	The therapist acts as a stabilizer as the patient pushes according to the command. Resistance may or may not be added to this pattern depending on the goal. The pattern is applied unilaterally on the affected side.

Bilateral Upper Extremity

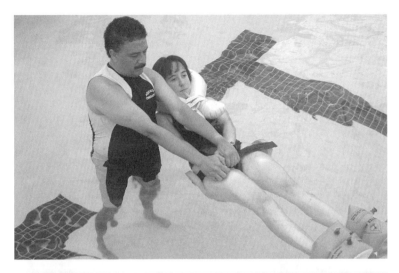

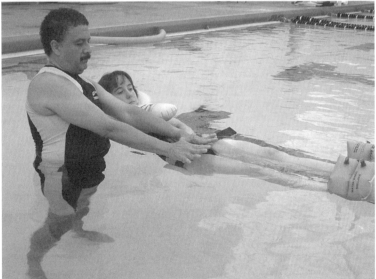

Figure 96: Bilateral upper extremity.

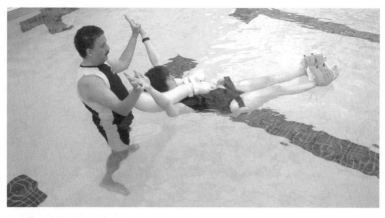

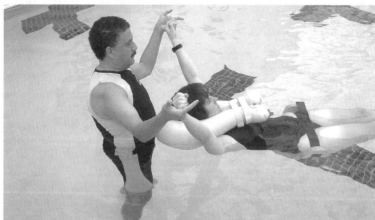

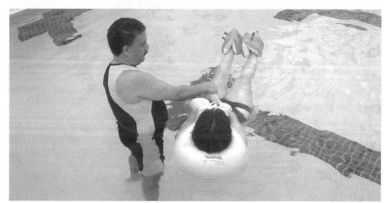

Figure 97: Bilateral upper extremity (continued).

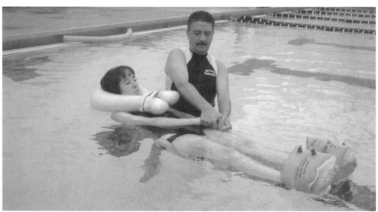

Figure 98: Bilateral upper extremity (continued).

Position of Patient	Supine wearing floatation collar, pelvic belt, and ankle rings. Both hands are placed on the left hip with shoulder internal rotation, forearm pronation, wrist and finger flexion bilaterally.
Position of Therapist	Standing on the patient's left side.
Hand Placement	The therapist's hands are placed on each of patient's fisted hands.
Command	"Keep your elbows straight. Open your fingers. Turn your palms up and push both arms out and back. Now, squeeze my hands making a fist. Turn your palms down and pull both arms down towards your right hip on the other side. Now let's repeat these same movements again so that we end up on the left side where we started."
Technique	The therapist stays in place while the patient moves from one side of the therapist to the other. This pattern can be applied with or without resistance.

Prone Unilateral Upper Extremity

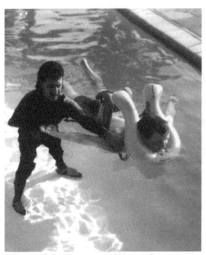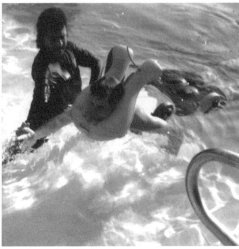

Figure 99: Prone unilateral upper extremity

Position of Patient	Prone wearing floatation cervical collar, pelvic belt, and a floatation noodle or belt at the chest. Mask and snorkel are optional. Both arms should be in shoulder extension, adduction, and internal rotation with forearm pronation, wrist, and finger flexion.
Position of Therapist	Standing by the affected side or extremity to be exercised.
Hand Placement	One hand is placed on the extensor surface of the patient's hand. The other hand stabilizes at the shoulder or scapular area.
Command	"Open your fingers. Turn your palm up and push your hand and arm up and overhead."
Technique	The patient pushes the arm up, out, and overhead. This can be an active-assistive pattern or resistance may be applied depending on the patient's clinical problem.

Indications and Contraindications

The following table provides information on specific clinical problems that warrant the use and application of the Bad Ragaz patterns and suggested contraindications:

Bad Ragaz Pattern	Indications	Contraindications
Passive Relaxation Position	• extensor spasticity • low back pain • sciatica	none
Passive Pelvic Tilt	• low back pain • sacroiliac joint dysfunction • degenerative lumbar disc disease • excessive anterior pelvic rotation • disc herniation	none
Passive Trunk Elongation with Pelvic Hold	• sacroiliac joint dysfunction • lumbar scoliosis • tight lumbodorsal fascia • asymmetrical hip levels • spasmodic erector spinae muscle • spasmodic intrinsic spine muscles • weak oblique muscles • rotated pelvis	status post-spinal fusion
Passive Trunk Elongation with Knee Hold	• tight quadratus lumborum muscle • decreased knee range of motion • knee joint pain • impaired knee joint proprioception • tight iliotibial band • weak gluteus medius • extensor spasticity	status post spinal fusion
Passive Trunk Elongation with Thoracic Hold	• tight scapular muscles • tight quadratus lumborum muscle • asymmetrical thoracic excursions with costovertebral and costotransverse involvement • weak intercostal muscles • weak oblique muscles	status post-spinal fusion
Passive Trunk Elongation with Elbow Hold	• weak latissimus dorsi and teres major muscles • tight pectoral girdle muscles • weak intercostal muscles • weak oblique muscles • tight scapular muscles • tight quadratus lumborum muscle	status post spinal fusion

Bad Ragaz Pattern	Indications	Contraindications
Isotonic #1	• weak abdominal muscles • lumbar spine arthropathy	tight hip flexors
Isotonic #2	• weak lateral trunk flexors • asymmetrical hip levels • tight lumbodorsal fascia	spasticity
Isometric	• weak hip extensor, knee extensor, ankle dorsiflexor, and hip adductor muscles • limited knee extension joint range • weak abdominal muscles	• fibromyalgia • polymyalgia • recurrent muscle spasms • spasticity
Tone Inhibition	• lower extremity extensor spasticity • decreased knee flexion • tight knee extensor muscles • tight knee joint ligaments	none
Pre-Weight-Bearing	• weak lower extremity flexor musculature • weak lower extremity extensor musculature • impaired kinesthesia and proprioception	extensor spasticity
Pre-Gait	• subtalar and mid-tarsal joint range limitations • fractures of the tarsals or metatarsals • weak dorsiflexor and plantar flexor muscles • impaired lower extremity coordination • weak intrinsic foot muscles	none
Unilateral Lower Extremity	• weak hip stabilizers: gluteus medius and minimus and adductor muscles • weak hip external/internal rotators • weak foot evertors/invertors	• tight or spasmodic hip external rotators • piriformis tightness • exercise caution applying this pattern in the presence of spasticity

Bad Ragaz Pattern	Indications	Contraindications
Bilateral Lower Extremity	• weak hip flexors, abductors, and external rotators • weak abdominal muscles • weak foot evertors • trunk instability • weak erector spinae	exercise caution if the hip external rotators are tight; modify the pattern
Bilateral Symmetrical Lower Extremity #1	• extensor spasticity • low back pain • disc herniation • sciatica • weak hip and knee flexors • weak ankle dorsiflexors • weak hip external rotators and abductors • lumbar radiculopathy	piriformis tightness
Bilateral Symmetrical Lower Extremity #2	• weak erector spinae • weak cervical extensors with instability • weak scapular retractors • weak plantar flexors • weak hip and knee extensors	• extensor spasticity • tight or spasmodic scapular and shoulder girdle muscles • tight or spasmodic cervical extensors
Bilateral Reciprocal Lower Extremity	• impaired lower extremity kinesthesia and proprioception • impaired lower extremity coordination • weak unilateral hip external rotators • weak knee flexors • decreased range of motion in knee flexion • decreased range of motion in hip external rotation • weak knee extensors	• piriformis syndrome • tight or spasmodic hip external rotators • tendency towards developing muscle cramps • intermittent claudication

Bad Ragaz Pattern	Indications	Contraindications
Unilateral Upper Extremity	<ul><li>weak rotator cuff muscles</li><li>weak shoulder abductor muscles</li><li>weak forearm pronators/supinators</li><li>weak pectoral girdle muscles</li><li>limited range of motion in shoulder abduction, external rotation, and forearm supination</li><li>impaired upper extremity coordination</li><li>impaired upper extremity proprioception</li><li>weak extensors of the fingers and intrinsics of the hand</li><li>weak wrist extensors</li></ul>	tendency towards recurrent dislocation of the shoulder joint
Bilateral Upper Extremity	<ul><li>weak rotator cuff muscles</li><li>weak shoulder abductor muscles</li><li>weak forearm pronators/supinators</li><li>weak pectoral girdle muscles</li><li>limited range of motion in shoulder abduction, external rotation, and forearm supination</li><li>impaired upper extremity coordination</li><li>impaired upper extremity proprioception</li><li>weak extensors of the fingers and intrinsics of the hand</li><li>weak wrist extensors and flexors</li><li>scapulohumeral instability with poor flexibility and mobility</li></ul>	tendency towards recurrent dislocation of the shoulder joint
Prone Unilateral Upper Extremity	<ul><li>flexor spasticity</li><li>weak unilateral scapular muscles</li><li>weak unilateral shoulder flexors</li><li>weak unilateral shoulder internal and external rotators</li><li>limited range of motion in shoulder flexion</li><li>weak finger flexors and extensors</li><li>weak wrist extensors and flexors</li></ul>	tendency towards recurrent dislocation of the shoulder joint

Conclusion

When deciding on the most effective pattern to use as part of the patient's plan of care, the aquatic therapist must focus on the patient's diagnosis, clinical problems, and clinical findings on the initial pre-aquatic evaluation. Limitations in range of motion, weakness of specific muscle groups, and other neurological deficits will set the stage for a prescriptive pattern that addresses the established clinical problems. Likewise, any precautions or contraindication must be carefully considered. Based on his applied knowledge of anatomy and pathophysiology, the aquatic therapist will be able to modify a particular pattern according to the patient's condition, tolerance, and limitations.

CHAPTER 5

APPLICATION OF WATSU®

What is Watsu®?

Watsu® is an applied intervention used in aquatic therapy which incorporates static passive stretches and a structured sequence of passive limb, head, and neck movements or patterns performed at water surface level. Watsu® was created by Harold Dull in Harbin Hot Springs, California. Based on the theories of meridians and energy flow, Watsu® introduces applied techniques of Zen Shiatsu into the water environment. Hence, its name "Watsu" which was intended to mean "water shiatsu." The primary objective of Watsu® is to allow the body to drift into a deeper state of relaxation. Because the patient is cradled by the practitioner at water surface level throughout the various movement sequences, weight is reduced from the vertebrae and extremities, thus enhancing muscle relaxation. Once relaxation is achieved and, aided by the weightlessness effects, spine flexibility is increased to levels far beyond what can be reached on land where we work against the force of gravity.

Clinical Objectives

Although the clinical relevance of Watsu® has not been fully established through scientific inquiry, outcomes described by therapists in case studies of patients with orthopedic and neurologic disorders seem to indicate that Watsu® can be potentially beneficial given the nature of the patient's clinical problems. Based on reported clinical outcomes, the following are potential physiologic effects derived from the application of Watsu®:

1. improvement in circulation
2. decrease in muscle fatigue
3. decrease in pain or tenderness
4. decrease in muscle tone
5. increase in range of motion

6. increase in spine or joint flexibility
7. improvement in tidal volume
8. improvement in postural alignment
9. resolution of muscle spasms
10. decrease in tension and stress
11. improvement in sleep patterns

Watsu® can also be described as a "nurturing" approach. As such, it can have potential emotional, psychological, and spiritual effects on the receiver. It is not uncommon for patients to experience an emotional release during or after a Watsu® session. Therefore, it is important for the practitioner to maintain a professional focus at all times and establish and maintain personal and professional boundaries.

When the patient reaches deeper states of relaxation, the levels of consciousness may be altered as well. This occurrence will depend on the patient's ability to surrender to the technique and on the practitioner's accuracy in performing each movement or sequence correctly. It is extremely important for the practitioner to monitor the patient's level of consciousness throughout the Watsu® session.

Guidelines

When considering Watsu® as a viable intervention in the aquatic rehabilitation plan of care, a number of precautions should be considered in order to optimize the therapeutic effects:

1. The optimal temperature of the water should be maintained between 90° to 92°F. The temperature should not exceed 94°F. Caution should be exercised for patients diagnosed with multiple sclerosis. In these cases, the temperature of the water must not exceed 90°F. For optimal results, the recommended temperature range for patients with multiple sclerosis is 88°F. The aquatic therapist must be well aware of the patient's history and related medical problems. If a musculoskeletal problem has been identified on the pre-aquatic evaluation, Watsu® might be beneficial, depending on the established goals and clinical objectives. If the patient suffers from an acute inflammatory condition, it is advised to wait until the condition has reached the subacute stages to begin the Watsu® sessions. When intervertebral discs are involved or when there is history of calcium loss (e.g., osteoporosis), caution should be taken in the application of certain movement sequences characterized by intense stretching of the soft and connective tissue. All in all, under these circumstances it would be strongly advised to obtain clearance from the patient's physician.

2. The degree of psychological dependency that the patient might exhibit could present a problem. Therefore, the practitioner must be well aware of the patient's limits and of his or her own limits as well.

3. The energy that is exchanged between the giver and the receiver during a Watsu® session creates an ambience of non-sexual intimacy. The aquatic therapist must be extremely careful and ethical in order to avoid overstepping the limits of intimacy.

4. The patient's cervical region must be supported at all times during a Watsu® session. Hyperextension must be avoided. A position of axial extension is ideal because it would assist in releasing tension and tightness of the suboccipital

muscles, the cervical extensors, and the ligamentum nuchae.

5. The patient's face (particularly the nose) must be kept above the water at all times. If possible, the patient should wear earplugs, particularly if there is a tendency to develop ear infections.

6. The practitioner should check the pH of the water. The aquatic therapist must document any reported susceptibility for allergic reactions to chemical agents such as bromine or chlorine.

7. The ideal water depth for an effective Watsu® session is three to four feet. Otherwise, the practitioner could lose control and support of the patient. Performing Watsu® in water depths exceeding four feet could potentially affect the therapist's body mechanics.

8. In order to avoid dehydration effects, both the practitioner and the patient should drink appropriate amounts of water prior to and after the Watsu® session.

9. The pool environment should be calm. A noisy environment would disrupt the flow of the session and interfere with the patient's ability to reach the desired level of relaxation. Soft instrumental or easy listening music is advised to enhance relaxation in a calm environment.

10. The practitioner must thoroughly explain to the patient the goals and outcomes to be achieved through the application of Watsu®, the specific movement sequences that will be used, and the rationale for their use. As a rule of ethics, the aquatic therapist must ask to be notified if the patient does not feel comfortable with any of the applied movements. Depending on the pa-

tient's response to the first Watsu® session, the therapist will be able to modify the session accordingly.

Contraindications

Identified problems that would contraindicate the application of Watsu® as an intervention in the aquatic plan of care are basically the same as those contraindicating the use of the pool for any other patient. The contraindications in the first list are referred to as absolute. These include, but are not limited to, the following:

1. active menstruation
2. uncontrolled bowel and bladder incontinence
3. skin infections (e.g., impetigo)
4. allergy to pool chemicals (e.g., chlorine, bromine)
5. severe vestibular problems (e.g., vertigo)
6. open wounds

Relative contraindications are those where the intervention might be performed observing certain modifications, precautions, and applications with clearance from the patient's physician. Among the relative contraindications, the following should be considered:

Total Hip Arthroplasty

On patients who have undergone a hip arthroplasty, excessive hip rotations (particularly internal rotation) and flexion should be avoided in order to prevent dislocation of the prosthetic hip. Hip flexion of 90° is usually allowed, but some physicians limit the flexion even more.

Status Post Spine Surgery

Spinal fusions present a contraindication for any passive movement that enhances spine mobility. In addition to clearance from the patient's physician, the aquatic therapist should exercise extreme caution when performing Watsu® with patients who are post laminectomy or discectomy. In these cases, a specially designed Watsu® program is allowed.

Basic Flow

The first sequence of movements is referred to as the "basic flow." The sequence that I present in this chapter under the category of "basic flow" movements differs for the one designed by Harold Dull in his original protocol. Another unique feature of the Watsu® protocol presented in this chapter is a change in the terminology that described the characteristic movements. The terminology used herein reflects a descriptive biomechanical pattern of movement.

Watsu® emphasizes the practice of coordinated deep breathing activities throughout the session. The session begins with the so-called "water breath dance." The water breath dance inte-

grates deep breathing with relaxation techniques. Both the therapist and the patient must assume the "cube" position (Figure 100). This position refers to a sitting position in shallow water with the hip flexed to approximately 90°, abducted to approximately 45°, and in slight external rotation. The knees are flexed to 90° and the feet should be in line with the direction of the patella. The patient should be instructed to "sit" on his pelvis. For patients who have a pronounced lordosis and anteriorly rotated pelvis, this might be difficult. If the patient is having difficulty aligning himself appropriately in the cube position, the therapist can teach him to perform a pelvic tilt in the sitting position. This would allow the degree of posterior pelvic rotation required for correct posture in the cube position.

At first, instruction on how to assume the cube position should begin with the patient's back against the wall. The patient should be taught to breathe in through the nose and out through the mouth. Relaxation begins with the water breath dance. As the patient begins to relax, the therapist should

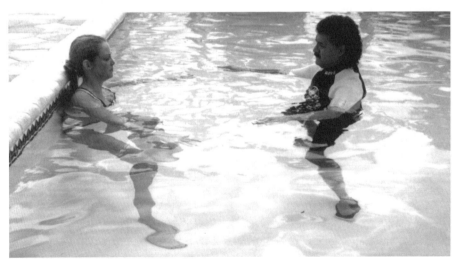

Figure 100: The "cube" position at the start of the water breath dance.

increase awareness of the buoyancy effects on the body through deep breathing exercises. Upon inspiratory effort, the patient's body will rise, while it tends to sink on expiration. It is important to indicate to the patient that when the session is coming to an end, he will be brought back to the starting point and will once again feel the wall against his back. When the patient feels that he is beginning to enter a stage of relaxation, he is instructed to walk away from the wall approximately three to four steps while maintaining the cube position.

The practitioner indicates that he will walk to the right of the patient, cradle the patient's head and neck on

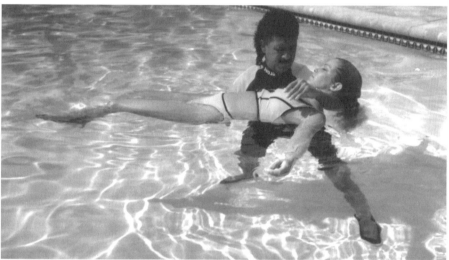

Figure 101: The head cradle.

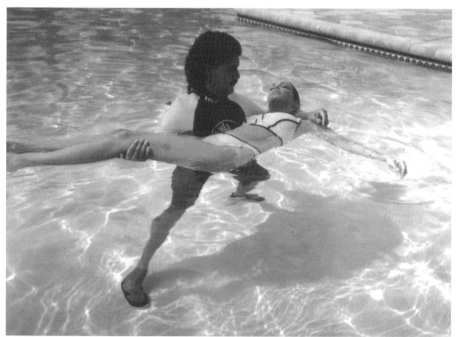

Figure 102: The "open arms" position.

the cubital fossa of his left arm, and bring the patient into a horizontal supine position. This is known as the *head cradle* (Figure 101). The dorsum of the practitioner's right hand is placed on the patient's sacrum with the knuckles positioned on the sacral sulcus. Once in this position, the body is allowed to flow freely and the practitioner can perform a series of snake-like movements to intensify the relaxation effects. When momentum is gained during the snake-like movements, the legs will swing and the popliteal surface of the patient's lower limbs will land on the therapist's right forearm in what is known as the *open arms* position (Figure 102).

This position permits the practitioner to perform the first sequence of movements beginning with the *bilateral repetitive lower extremity flexor-extensor pattern* (Figure 103) originally called the accordion. This movement accentuates hip and knee flexion with synchronous lumbar-pelvic rhythm performed in a passive knee-to-chest pattern. It is important to coordinate the movement with the patient's breathing pattern, that is, when the patient exhales the flexion component takes place and, vice versa, the extension component coincides with inhalation.

The repetitive flexor-extensor pattern gradually leads to the *bilateral repetitive lower extremity rotational flexor-extensor pattern* (Figure 104). This was called the rotating accordion in the original sequence. The knees are the landmarks of reference in this movement because they are rotated in a counterclockwise direction. The patient's deep breathing pattern continues to be coordinated with the various aspects of the movement. Additionally, the therapist should perform the rotational movements in a rhythmical manner observing proper body mechanics.

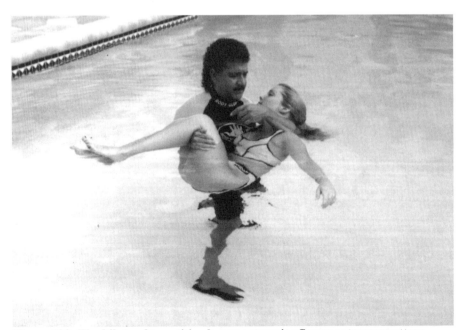

Figure 103: The bilateral repetitive lower extremity flexor-extensor pattern.

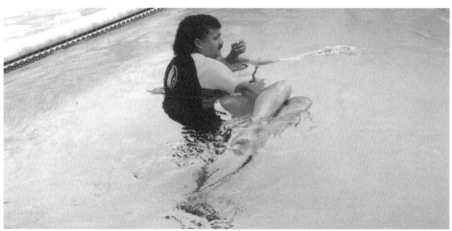

Figure 104: The bilateral repetitive lower extremity rotational flexor-extensor pattern.

Gradually, the practitioner drops the far leg but continues to rotate the near leg. This movement involves *unilateral hip and knee flexion with rotation* (Figure 105) and was originally referred to as the near leg rotation. This sequence of movements leading up to and including the unilateral flexion with rotation pattern not only focuses on increasing joint flexibility with mobility but additionally contributes to hypotonicity in cases where spasticity is a clinical problem.

The sequence moves subsequently into the so-called *capture* (Figure 106). The capture sequence presented in this chapter follows the original format described by Harold Dull.

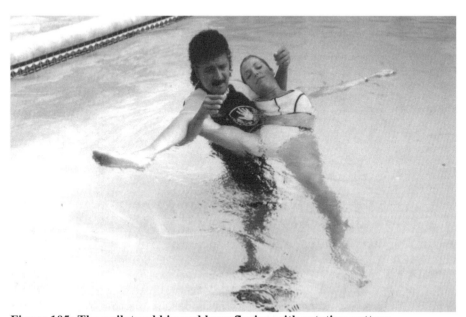

Figure 105: The unilateral hip and knee flexion with rotation pattern.

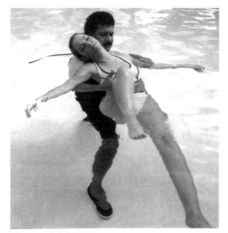

Figure 106: The capture.

The practitioner's left hand holds the patient's occiput and upper cervical region while the right hand is holding the popliteal surface of the near knee. The next step towards achieving the capture involves flexing the patient's hip and bringing the head towards the knee. At the same time, the patient is moved away from the practitioner while he is turned so that his head will end up resting on the practitioner's right shoulder. In this position, the practitioner

performs *alternate contralateral passive stretches to the shoulder adductors, shoulder flexors, hip extensors, and hip adductors* (Figure 107 and Figure 108). This movement has been descriptively called the arm-leg rock. At the shoulder, the stretched muscles are the pectoralis major and minor, the anterior deltoid, and the coracobrachialis. Because of the position of the patient, the latissimus dorsi is not affected in this passive stretch. In the lower extremity, the gluteus maximus, the pectineus, the gracilis, and the adductor magnus, longus, and brevis figure among the muscles stretched. The adductor group of hip muscles are particularly stretched proximally. The contralateral alternate passive stretches are also synchronized with the patient's deep breathing pattern.

While maintaining hold of the patient's right knee, the therapist passes that knee on to his left hand, places his right hand over the patient's right

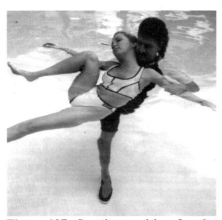

Figure 107: Starting position for the contralateral passive stretch technique to the shoulder adductors, shoulder flexors, hip extensors, and hip adductors.

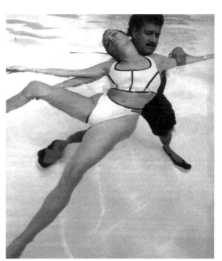

Figure 108: Ending position for the contralateral passive stretch technique to the shoulder adductors, shoulder flexors, hip extensors, and hip adductors.

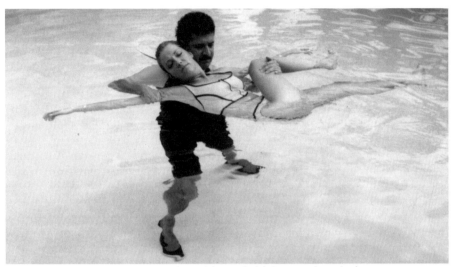

Figure 109: The sustained trunk and lateral thigh stretch technique.

shoulder and twists the upper and lower halves of the body in two different directions. This is called the *sustained trunk and lateral thigh stretch* (Figure 109). The structures affected by this stretch are the anterolateral abdominal muscles, the iliotibial band, the lumbodorsal fascia, and the horizontal shoulder adductors on the right side.

Once again, the practitioner's hand now holds the patient's head at the occiput while the left hand is holding

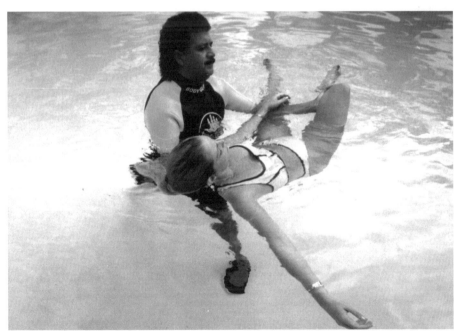

Figure 110: Atlantoaxial and lumbosacral joint rotation.

the knee at the popliteal surface. The sequential pattern that began with the capture and continued on to the alternate contralateral stretch and static trunk stretch now places the practitioner on the opposite side of the patient. In this position, the aquatic therapist begins to rock the patient back and forth.

This particular movement consists of stepping forward with one leg and backwards with the opposite leg while maintaining a static position of the arms. The hand-held points, that is, the head and knee do not move. Instead the thigh, pelvis, and spine will rotate in an axis around the hand-held points of reference. The movement is meant to elicit an *atlantoaxial and lumbosacral joint rotation* (Figure 110) and has been called the knee-head rock. After a series of rocking motions, a few seconds of stillness follow. The dorsum of the practitioner's left hand is then placed on the patient's sacrum as he proceeds to perform *lateral sacral glides with coordinated side-to-side cervical rotations* (Figure 111) in opposite directions. This free movement consists of rocking the sacrum causing mobilizations of the sacroiliac joint and at the same time facilitating free-flowing cervical rotations.

Gradually, the patient's head is placed on the therapist's left shoulder. The therapist will hold the patient's hips bilaterally with the thumbs pointing to the anterior superior iliac spines and begins to push one hip down with a simultaneous backward sweep of the hips and extended legs. This movement involves an *alternate transverse pelvic and sacroiliac joint rotation with lateral tilt* (Figure 112). Its original name is the hip rock.

In order to return to the original position, the practitioner holds the patient's right hip with his left hand and reaches for the patient's right arm with his right hand. Once he is holding the patient's right arm, the practitioner threads the arm through his left arm and frees the arms allowing him to assume the head cradle position again. This technique concludes the basic flow sequence.

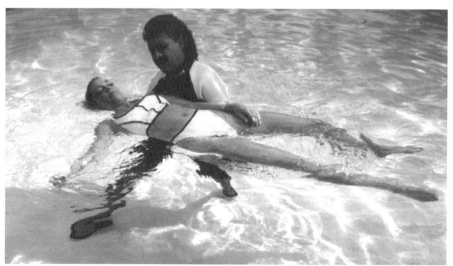

Figure 111: The lateral sacral glide technique with coordinated cervical rotations.

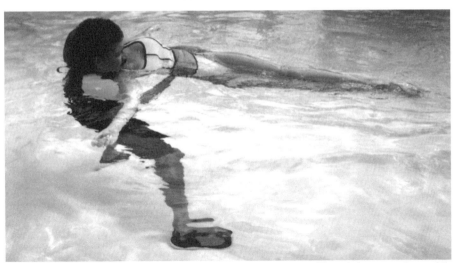

Figure 112: The alternate transverse pelvic and sacroiliac joint rotation with lateral tilt pattern.

Transitional Flow

As the transitional flow sequence begins, the first three movement sequences are performed. In addition to rotating the near leg, the far leg is also passively rotated. This technique allows the therapist to move his hand towards the ankle on the far leg and proceed to flex the hip and knee above the water until he is able to pass the leg over his head and rest it on the back of his neck.

Commonly called the "far leg over," this movement consists of *full*

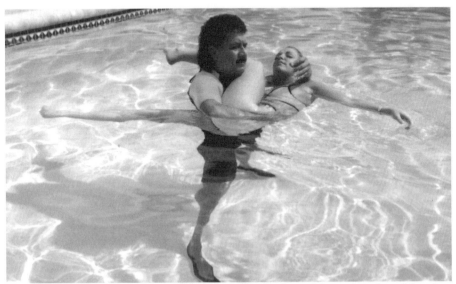

Figure 113: The full range contralateral hip flexion with a gluteal and lumbar soft tissue stretch technique.

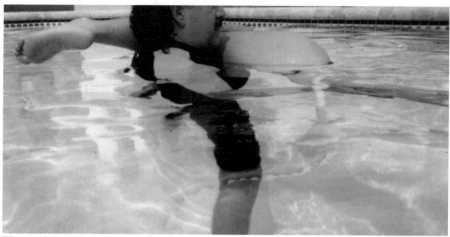

Figure 114: The sustained hip flexor stretch technique.

range contralateral hip flexion with a gluteal and lumbar soft tissue stretch (Figure 113). While maintaining this position, the therapist will perform a *sustained hip flexor stretch* (Figure 114) on the extended leg. This technique was originally known as the "leg push." The static stretch is sustained for a few seconds. The extended leg is flexed at the hip and knee and placed over the practitioner's abdomen allowing him to perform a *caudal sacrum glide* (Figure 115) or sacrum pull. The subtalar and midtarsal joints can also be passively ranged while working on the extended lower extremity. Gentle pétrissage can be applied to the gastrocsoleus muscle.

Thereafter, this same leg is swung over to the other side. While the thera-

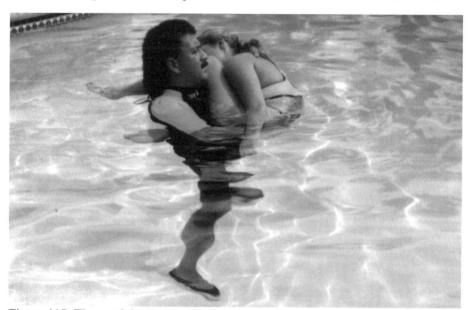

Figure 115: The caudal sacrum glide technique.

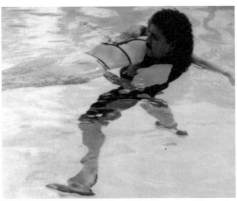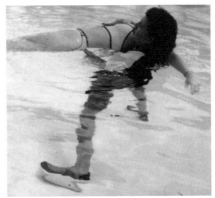

Figure 116: The sternal compression technique with alternate caudal sacral glide.

pist maintains hold of the metacenter at T11, one hand moves under the patient's neck and over the opposite shoulder and finally rests on the patient's sternum. The heel of the opposite hand is placed on the patient's sacrum. *Sternal compressions with alternate caudal sacral glides* (Figure 116) are performed. This movement was initially called the spine lengthening technique. Sternal compressions are performed on exhalation while sacral glides are performed on inhalation. This technique seems to be particularly

beneficial for patients suffering from sacroiliac joint displacement.

Having transferred one hand to the occiput while the other hand is maintained at the sacrum, a single spine pull or distraction of the spine in opposite direction follows as the next movement. This is called *cervico-lumbar distraction* (Figure 117) and is applied by pulling the occiput in the direction of the head and the sacrum in the direction of the feet. The distraction is sustained for several seconds. With one hand still placed on the sacrum, an undulating

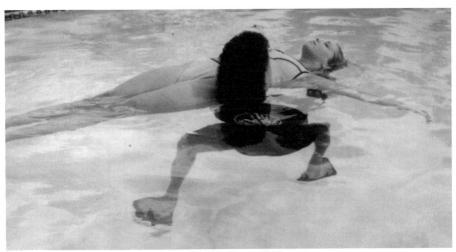

Figure 117: The cervico-lumbar distraction technique.

spine movement is performed consisting of upward thrusts of the sacrum. Biomechanically, this is referred to as *anterior sacral glides* (Figure 118). The force that causes the glide of the sacrum does not originate on the practitioner's arm or hand. Instead, it originates from repetitive bilateral plantar flexion movements, which, in turn, elicits an undulating wavelike movement of the pelvis and trunk, which subsequently result in the sacral thrust. This concludes the transitional flow of patterns and movements.

In order to assume the original open arms position, the therapist must hold the patient's arm at 90° of shoulder abduction with his right hand while the left hand moves up to hold the occiput. The patient is moved through the buoyancy of the water. When momentum is gained, the head is cradled and the legs are held at the popliteal surfaces. Several bilateral repetitive flexor-extensor patterns are performed as the patient is returned to the wall where it all started. It is important to stabilize or anchor the patient's back against the wall. Stabilizing the head is another important consideration particularly if the patient has

drifted into a state of optimal relaxation. Gently, the practitioner should distance himself from the patient and wait for a reaction indicating recovery.

Arthrokinematics and Soft Tissue Structures

This section will discuss the biomechanical components of characteristic movements featured in the Watsu® basic and transitional flows. The analysis presented in this section is a comprehensive arthrokinematic dissection of movements and their effect on articular structures, muscles, and ligaments. I maintain that acquiring a practical knowledge of the biomechanical foundations of Watsu® will empower the aquatic therapist with applied expertise on concave-convex joint surface relationships and their impact on connective as well as muscular tissue. Consequently, it allows the clinician to be more selective in the integration of Watsu® as a viable intervention in the patient's aquatic plan of care based on established short- and long-term goals and the identified clinical problems.

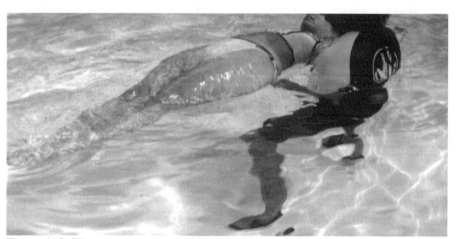

Figure 118: The anterior sacral glide technique.

The movements discussed in this section will retain the designated biomechanical terminology or an abbreviated term. The terms "ipsilateral" and "contralateral" are used frequently in this discussion. I refer to "ipsilateral" as the extremity closest to or the same side as the practitioner. "Contralateral" implies that the technique is applied on the extremity farthest from or on the opposite side of the therapist.

Bilateral Repetitive Lower Extremity Flexor-Extensor Pattern

This movement is divided in two phases: the flexor phase and the extensor phase. As discussed previously in this chapter, the flexor phase is coordinated with the expiratory phase of breathing. The extensor phase is performed with inspiration. Therefore, the diaphragmatic dome is elevated to its resting position during the flexor phase. Flexion and extension are movements that occur in the sagittal plane of progression around a transverse axis.

The hip joint will flex to approximately 150° producing a passive stretch on the iliolumbar fascia, the gluteus maximus muscle, the ligamenta flava of the lumbar vertebrae, and two of the components of the erector spinae muscle, the longissimus lumborum and the spinalis lumborum. During the flexor phase of this movement, the femoral head rotates posteriorly on the acetabulum. This is a convex on concave articular motion, which can also be interpreted conversely, that is, the acetabulum rotates anterior on the femoral head.

The considerable amount of bilateral hip flexion that takes place will facilitate a posterior tilt of the os coxae on the sacrum causing a passive stretch to the sacroiliac ligament. A chain reaction is elicited with flexion of the lumbar spine. This sequence of multiarticular movements that are interdependent on each other is known as the lumbar-pelvic rhythm. In this case, it is an open-chain phenomenon, which recruits the acetabulofemoral, sacroiliac, and lumbar zygapophyseal joints contributing to an increase in the range of motion of these joints and at the same time improving the function of the structures affected. The deep intrinsic layer of lumbar spine muscles consisting of the intertransversarii, multifidi, and interspinous muscles are also passively stretched during the flexor phase of this movement.

The cradle position of the receiver permits a certain amount of cervical spine flexion. Consequently, the ligamentum nuchae, splenius capitis muscle, semispinalis capitis muscle, suboccipital muscles, levator scapulae muscle, and the superior fibers of the upper trapezius are among the soft and connective tissue structures affected.

In the extensor phase, there is not complete hip extension to the 0° position. Instead, the hip joint is maintained at approximately -20° of extension. Because of the proximal insertion, the iliopsoas and pectineus muscles will sustain some degree of passive stretch during this phase.

All spinal segments (cervical, thoracic, and lumbar) will extend. This will produce a stretch on the rectus abdominis muscle, the internal and external oblique muscles, and the intercostal musculature.

Bilateral Repetitive Lower Extremity Rotational Flexor-Extensor Pattern

The rotating accordion, as it is commonly referred to, involves a simultaneous yet alternating internal rotation with flexion of the ipsilateral hip with external rotation and flexion of the contralateral hip. The movement performed is a counterclockwise circular movement, which occurs on a transverse plane around a longitudinal axis. Two biomechanical considerations apply in this case:

1. The ipsilateral femoral head rotates medially and posteriorly producing a passive stretch to the iliotibial band, the ischiofemoral ligament, the gluteus medius muscle, the piriformis muscle, and the other five external rotators of the hip.
2. The contralateral femoral head rotates anteriorly and laterally producing a passive stretch of the Y Ligament of Bigelow (also known as the iliofemoral ligament) and the pubofemoral ligament.

The degrees of bilateral hip flexion can range from 90° to 110° and will stretch the gluteus maximus muscle.

Unilateral Hip and Knee Flexion with Rotation

The components of this movement occur in three planes: coronal, sagittal, and transverse. With the exception of the rotational elements, the sequence of movements mirrors the arthrokinematics of both the accordion and rotating accordion with the same estimated degrees of hip flexion and the same anatomical structures affected.

This particular movement divides into three phases. The first is the flexor phase, which is identical to the accordion movement. The second phase has two components:

1. External rotation with abduction where the femoral head rotates anteriorly and laterally on a longitudinal axis. This rotation passively stretches the muscular structures on the anteromedial aspect of the thigh. These include the tensor fascia latae, the adductor magnus, the

adductor longus, the adductor brevis, the gracilis muscle, and the pectineus. Additionally, two ligaments are affected, the iliofemoral and the pubofemoral.
2. Internal rotation with abduction where the femoral head rotates posteriorly and medially on a longitudinal axis stretching such structures as the gluteus medius and minimus muscles, the iliotibial band (IT), the piriformis muscle, and two ligaments of the posterior gluteal and sacral regions, the sacrotuberous and sacrospinous ligaments.

Finally, the third phase consists of extension of the hip to -20°, a motion that will affect the superficial hip flexors as well as the proximal anteromedial hip ligaments.

Alternate Contralateral Passive Stretches to the Shoulder Adductors, Shoulder Flexors, Hip Extensors, and Hip Adductors

This is a passive movement of the ipsilateral shoulder with simultaneous passive range of motion of the contralateral hip and knee. Shoulder abduction occurs on a coronal plane around an anteroposterior axis. Scapulothoracic motions complement the scapulohumeral rhythm produced with integrated movement of the acromioclavicular and sternoclavicular joints. Scapular movements are effectuated on a frontal plane around an anteroposterior axis.

Two phases characterize this movement. The first phase consists of abduction of the contralateral shoulder to 120° with a few degrees of external rotation. During this movement, a passive stretch to the pectoral muscles, the coracobrachialis, and teres major muscle, and the glenohumeral ligament is produced. Additionally, there are two scapulothoracic contributions: scapular upward rotation with retraction, which will stretch the lower trapezius and rhomboid major muscles, and elevation of the acromioclavicular joint with depression and rotation of the sterno-clavicular joint with impact on the acromioclavicular, coracoclavicular, and sternoclavicular ligaments.

The second phase involves a com-bination of movements that occur in the sagittal and coronal planes of progres-sion with rotating axes. These move-ments begin with flexion of the contra-lateral hip to 135° followed by flexion of the knee to 150° and hip abduction to 35° with external rotation to 40°. The following anatomical structures sustain a passive stretch in the second phase of this "contralateral stretch" pattern:
1. gluteus maximus muscle
2. gracilis muscle
3. adductor magnus muscle
4. adductor longus muscle
5. adductor brevis muscle
6. pectineus muscle
7. sacrotuberous ligament
8. sacrospinous ligament

Sustained Trunk and Lateral Thigh Stretch

This is a simultaneous passive stretch where the ipsilateral hip and shoulder are moved in opposite direc-tions. It is another movement high-lighted by two components. The first phase consists of hip flexion to 100° and approximately 45° of passive internal rotation. This twisting maneu-ver will cause a passive stretch to the quadratus lumborum and piriformis muscles, iliocostalis lumborum compo-nent of the erector spinae, lumbar multifidi, and rotatores. The sacroiliac ligaments as well as the iliotibial band are also stretched. In the second half of

the movement, there are approximately 10° to 25° of shoulder hyperextension with a few degrees of external rotation causing an effect on the shoulder girdle with emphasis on the pectoral and shoulder muscles particularly the inter-nal rotators and flexors. Due to the fact that the thoracic cage will also be involved in the movement, the inter-costal muscles will be affected as well. Ligamentous involvement includes the coracohumeral and glenohumeral ligaments.

Atlantoaxial and Lumbosacral Joint Rotation

The dens of the axis articulates with the posterior articular facet of the arch of the atlas. This rotation is ac-centuated in this movement. Inferiorly, the same rotational movement takes place between L5 and S1.

Lateral Sacral Glides with Coordinated Side-to-Side Cervical Rotations

It is more appropriate to think of this movement as freeing the sacrum but in the process a passive rotation of all spine segments is facilitated biome-chanically. Based on the principles of kinesiology, all rotation occurs on a transverse plane around a longitudinal axis. An analysis of this motion will demonstrate that the upper spine re-gions (cervical and thoracic) will move in an opposite direction to the lower spine regions (lumbar and sacrum), thus stretching the intrinsic rotatores mus-cles.

Alternate Transverse Pelvic and Sacroiliac Joint Rotation with Lateral Tilt

In the first part of this movement both os coxae are rotated transversely around the sacrum. The right hip is rotated down towards the water and posteriorly on the sacroiliac joint while the left hip moves up. Subsequently, since the sartorius muscle originates in the anterior superior iliac spine (ASIS), it will undergo a passive stretch. However, the greatest impact occurs in the ligamentous structure protecting the sacroiliac region and the anterior acetabulofemoral area.

The second part of the pattern reflects a backward swing of both lower extremities stretching the hamstring muscles at their origin in the ischial tuberosity as well as the ligaments that protect the inferior gluteal region, the sacrotuberous and sacrospinous ligaments.

Full Range Contralateral Hip Flexion with a Gluteal and Lumbar Soft Tissue Stretch

Traditionally, this movement was referred to as the "far leg over" because the contralateral leg was lifted and positioned to rest over the therapist's neck. This position allows a stretch of the contralateral hip extensors (gluteus maximus) and lumbosacral structures. Because of its anatomical location largely related to origin and insertion, there is an additional release of the piriformis muscle through the applied stretch. The interjected term "full" has been appropriately given and implies maximal range of hip flexion to approximately 150° or higher.

As the movement of the contralateral leg progresses, the femoral head rotates internally stretching the sacrospinous and sacrotuberous ligaments. When the popliteal surface of the far knee is resting on the extensor surface of the practitioner's neck, the knee is flexed to approximately 150°, which will increase the passive tension on the patellar ligament and moderately on the iliotibial band. Additionally, there will be some degree of lumbar spine flexion placing the ligamentum flavia in a stretched position. As the lumbar spine flexes, the pelvis goes into a posterior tilt. This posterior pelvic tilt will release the thoracolumbar myofascia and any hyperactivity of the type Ia and II fibers of the erector spinae and intrinsic deep layer muscles of the lumbar region.

Sustained Hip Flexor Stretch

While the contralateral leg is maintained in the stretched position, both the superficial and deep hip flexors of the opposite leg are manually stretched by pushing the thigh into hyperextension approximately 15° to 20°. The superficial hip flexors are the sartorius and tensor fascia latae. The deep hip flexor is the iliopsoas but the rectus femoris at its origin is said to be a synergist in this movement when there is mechanical disadvantage of its function at the knee joint.

Caudal Sacrum Glide

The sacrum glide is best performed with the patient's leg placed over the practitioner's abdomen. This position gives the practitioner a more accurate hand placement and control of the sacrum. The tips of the index finger and thumb should be placed at the ala of the sacrum or at the superior sacroarticular facets. When proper grip takes place, distraction of the sacrum occurs by manually separating the sacral promontory and the vertebral body of the fifth lumbar vertebrae. The articular distraction that occurs in the lumbosacral region stretches both the iliolumbar ligament and the posterior longitudinal ligament.

Sternal Compressions with Alternate Caudal Sacral Glides

This movement figures among those that have been described as having a dual component. The first phase involves the application of sternal compressions, which will produce trunk and hip flexion aided by the effects of buoyancy. Performed during exhalation, sternal compressions are meant to strengthen the patient's vital capacity. The second phase will facilitate the antagonistic motions. However, there is additional distraction at the lumbosacral junction producing the same effects as the previously discussed technique.

Cervico-lumbar Distraction

This applied technique is described as a cephalocaudal distraction of the vertebral column. The hand that is holding the occiput will move in the direction of the head causing distraction of the cervical spine while the hand that holds the sacrum will move in the direction of the feet causing distraction at the lumbosacral area.

At the cervical region, the effects of the distraction will be higher at the atlanto-occipital and antantoaxial joints. Consequently, the following structures will be maximally stretched:
1. suboccipital muscles
2. tectorial membrane
3. interspinous ligaments
4. intertransverse ligaments
5. anterior longitudinal ligament
6. posterior longitudinal ligament
7. ligamentum nuchae
8. splenius capitis
9. splenius cervicis
10. ligamentum flava

The upper trapezius, levator scapulae, and sternocleidomastoid muscles will sustain a moderate stretch but the effect will not be as intense as those felt suboccipitally. The cervical portion of the three components of the erector spinae might be minimally affected as well as the semispinalis capitis muscle.

At the lumbosacral region, the same described outcomes will be experienced in ligaments, myofascia, and some soft tissue structures such as the iliocostalis lumborum and the deep layer intrinsic lumbar musculature.

Anterior Sacral Glides

This technique consists of an applied mobilization of the sacrum anteriorly on its adjoining two innominate bones. The mobilization force is initiated with the motions of the talocrural joint in the legs, not in the hands. It is a force that is transferred to the thenar and hypothenar eminences of the hands, which are placed on the median sacral crest. The degree of mobilization produced will release the sacroiliac joint and reduce tension on the adjoining connective tissue structures. It is considered beneficial in patients suffering from sacroiliac joint disorders.

The wave of undulating motions tends to radiate to the lumbar, thoracic, and cervical spine. As a result the zygapophyseal joints will be indirectly or moderately affected, as will other associated soft and connective tissue structures in these anatomical regions.

Conclusion

The benefits derived from the clinical application of Watsu® in aquatic therapy are linked to the integration of passive stretches to the soft, myofascial, and connective tissue as well as the passive articular maneuvers that biomechanically characterize the described movements.

Through applied stretch-reflex facilitation, the techniques that incorporate passive stretches will strengthen the contractility of muscle fibers leading to an improved overall function of the motor unit. Likewise, if ligaments are stretched, the plastic deformation properties of the connective tissue will be maintained, thereby improving flexibility and stability. Finally, the arthrokinematic effects of Watsu® must be stressed. All the movement sequences and applied techniques featured in the protocol discussed in this chapter consist of either partial or full passive joint range of motion. The objective is to improve joint congruency and convex on concave articular dynamics.

CHAPTER 6
ADAPTING THE HALLIWICK METHOD

Introduction and Historical Perspective

The Halliwick Method was developed by James McMillan in 1949 at the Halliwick School for Girls in London, England. Initially, this method focused on swimming instruction and training. It later was developed and further structured into what is now a clinical approach used in the treatment of many types of physical impairments. The method supports the scientific principles of hydrodynamics and body mechanics, which accounts for its use as an aquatic therapy intervention.

The Halliwick Method provides patients with the opportunity to visualize themselves as independent and to set goals for themselves with the objective of regaining their functional independence. It serves as an incentive for patients boosting their self-confidence. The control of balance and subsequent correction of balance deficits has become a primary objective in the application of Halliwick techniques.

The basic philosophy of this approach revolves around the theories of balance control, motor control, and developmental maturation stages in the human being. Clinically speaking, this is the core of the Halliwick theory. Therefore, the clinical objectives, which have served as the basis for the introduction of the Halliwick Method into the aquatic rehabilitation arena, include:

1. improvement of muscle strength
2. improvement of motor control in the trunk and extremities
3. improvement of circulation
4. improvement of breathing patterns
5. improvement of static and dynamic balance
6. improvement of gait pattern
7. improvement of postural tone

These objectives have established the clinical relevance of Halliwick as a viable intervention popularly used in pediatrics. Halliwick does not employ the use of floatation devices in its techniques. Correct handling of the patient is another important consideration because it allows mobility and facilitates the expected movement or response to the activity.

Four Phases of Halliwick

The Halliwick Method consists of a series of activities, which have been grouped into four phases:

Phase I – Adjustment to the Aquatic Environment

This phase emphasizes the adjustment of the patient to the aquatic environment. As the patient becomes more comfortable in the water, he will acquire more freedom of movement. In doing so, the patient avoids working against the buoyancy effects. The "sit to crawl to kneel to stand" developmental sequence is reversed in this first phase of the Halliwick Method or when teaching anyone to swim. Therefore, activities in this phase are performed in the vertical position. In the subsequent phases, the patient will be placed in buoyant positions for more complex techniques.

Phase II – Rotations

In the second phase, position changes and body rotations are integrated. Sagittal and horizontal plane rotations are emphasized. One of the most practiced techniques is the "vertical to horizontal to vertical rotation" (Figure 119). The water is the medium that will hold the body buoyant once the horizontal position is assumed. This rotational activity is first practiced with guidance, but gradually the contact from the therapist is reduced as the patient learns to become more independent. The rotation of the body can follow a forward or backward direction, that is, the lower extremities may move forward while the head moves back or vice versa. If the body rotates in a forward direction, a mask and snorkel tube may be used. If the body rotates in a backward direction, no equipment is necessary. The therapist's hands are only used to enhance balance and provide support or control when necessary.

Vertical rotation around a horizontal axis is another phase II activity (Figure 120). It involves a 360° rotation of the entire body where the head leads the movement. The trunk and lower extremities follow until the rotation is completed. This technique can be

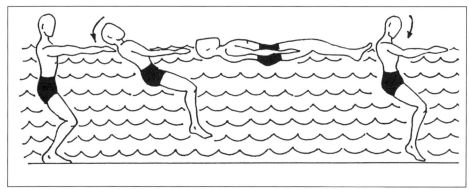

Figure 119: Vertical to horizontal to vertical rotations.

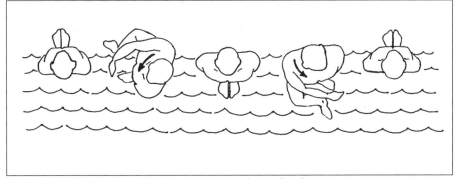

Figure 120: Vertical rotations around a horizontal axis.

practiced in shallow or deep water. It is often referred to as lateral rotation. It has been a useful strategy to teach patients to achieve independent entry into the water. However, this technique is not appropriate for patients with vestibular disorders.

Phase III – Control of Movement in the Water

In this phase the degree of control depends on whether or not the balanced position is maintained vertically, allowing the body to float. Integrated activities and techniques in this third phase are meant to challenge balance in a buoyant state.

Picking up objects from the bottom of the pool is a popular activity. The therapist uses objects that sink to the bottom of the pool and the patient is instructed to pick up these objects. The

activity begins in the standing position and progresses to a forward 180° rotation of the body where the head and upper extremities lead (Figure 121). In cases of upper extremity monoplegia, hypotonicity, weakness, or even hypertonicity, the patient should be encouraged to pick up the object with his weak hand.

Turbulent gliding is another featured activity. Aided by the effects of buoyancy, this activity induces balance and enhances control of body movement in the water (Figure 122). While maintained buoyant, the patient's body is moved passively by the aquatic therapist through the water as he creates turbulence at the head of the patient.

Phase IV – Freedom of Movement

Because of my intent to be more descriptive, I have renamed this phase.

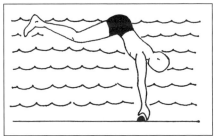

Figure 121: The patient picks up objects from the bottom of the pool.

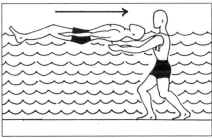

Figure 122: Floating balance control in the supine position.

The objective of phase IV is to achieve freedom of movement in the water. This is accomplished through active short-arc movements. Depending on the patient's capabilities and/or deficits, he can perform the activity using both arms in either the prone or supine positions. The activity can progress to a back crawl involving alternate rhythmical movements of both arms. The concept of the metacenter and Bernoulli's law are the foundations for phase IV Halliwick activities.

Kangaroo jumps figure among the more complex popular activities featured in this fourth phase (Figure 123). In the vertical or standing position, the patient's hand should be resting on the therapist's hand, that is, palm on palm. No gripping should be allowed, as this will only increase tension. The patient is instructed to jump, while maintaining stability and balance. Palm on palm contact is maintained at all times. This activity helps to restore dynamic balance for patients with balance deficits. Depending on the extent of balance disorder, the patient may be unable to perform kangaroo jumps. Simple ambulatory activity may be substituted.

The "bicycle ride" allows active lower extremity cyclical activity with support by the therapist (Figure 124).

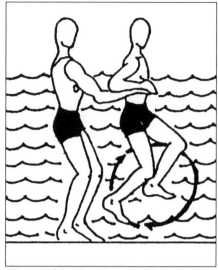

Figure 124: The bicycle ride activity.

The patient should keep his head forward over the knees and feet while being lifted and performing the bicycling motions. The patient's forearm rests upon the therapist's forearm. The therapist holds the patient's hand. This activity is useful as a reeducation technique.

In the "horizontal hold" activity (Figure 125), the therapist's hands are placed at the center of buoyancy. The patient can be maintained motionless or he can be instructed to move his legs in a "knee-to-chest pattern" or a "frog-kick pattern."

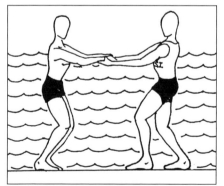

Figure 123: The position for the kangaroo jumps.

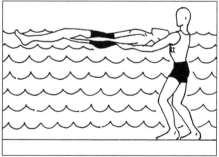

Figure 125: The horizontal hold activity.

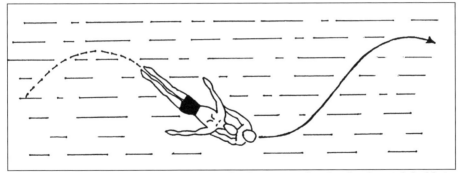

Figure 126: Passive movement through the water in the horizontal hold to induce relaxation.

These active, lower-extremity, integrated movements are helpful particularly in cases of lower extremity extensor spasticity or when there is evidence of associated back pain. A motionless horizontal hold is used when the goal is to induce relaxation. The patient is passively moved through the water in S-shaped curves (Figure 126). This has been referred to as "wriggling around the rock." If the therapist encounters difficulty with hand placement, body mechanics, and control of the patient in the horizontal supine

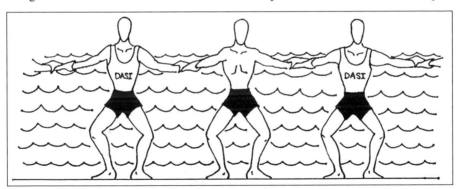

Figure 127: The long-arm hold technique.

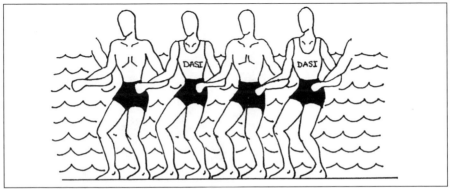

Figure 128: The short-arm hold technique.

position, the hands may be switched to each side of the patient's waist. Besides optimizing relaxation, this activity alternately stretches the lateral muscles and structures of the hip, thigh, and leg. The lateral effects of these movements on the hips may be potentially advantageous in sacroiliac joint problems.

Finally, group activities are another integral consideration in phase IV Halliwick. To ensure and maintain stability and safety, one of two techniques are always applied: the long-arm hold (Figure 127) and the short-arm hold (Figure 128). The applied use of either technique depends on the condition of the patient or the extent of clinical problems or identified deficits. If the aquatic therapist is working on one patient individually, the arm hold techniques will allow the therapist to have steadier control of the patient. Side-stepping gait or crab walk may be integrated. If group activities are performed, patients can form a circle or line.

Halliwick Applications

There are two applied movements that will maintain control of the body, balance, buoyancy, and efficient performance in the various positions described in the Halliwick Method. These are breathing control and chin control. They are considered the key to effective and efficient performance of Halliwick activities, particularly the rotations in phase II.

In order to achieve proper breathing control, a basic exercise involves the use of the so-called Halliwick blow-balls. These are spherical objects with a flattened ring in the center around the circumference. They have different colors on each side and float on the water. The patient is instructed to blow on the floating plastic balls and flip them 180° in order to show the opposite color (Figure 129). The emphasis of this exercise is on the improvement of tidal volume and vital capacity. The activity is practiced in shallow water.

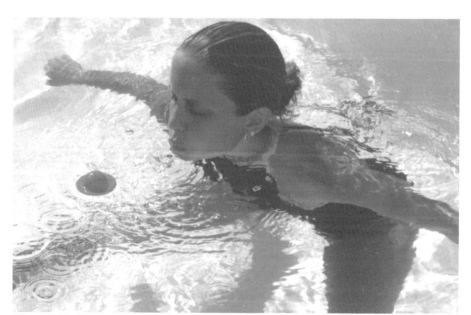

Figure 129: Integrated breathing control techniques using the flip balls.

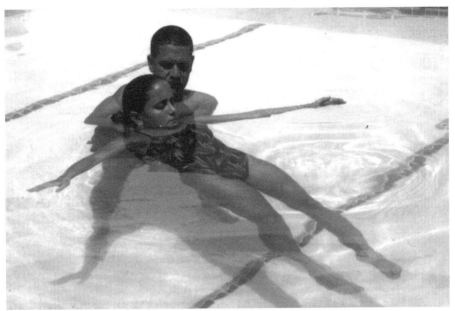

Figure 130: Integrated chin control techniques.

Chin control is essential, especially for activities that require sagittal and horizontal rotations of the body, control of movement, and free movement in the water. In rotational activities, the integration of chin control allows the patient to perform the movement as accurately as possible without associated compensatory motions. Therefore, proper practice of chin control will result in better motor control of the trunk musculature. In order to maintain balance and alignment in the vertical upright position in deep water, the patient should be instructed to use his chin to guide the movement. When the chin is depressed or moves towards the neck, the body will have a tendency to assume a prone recumbent position in the water (Figure 130). Conversely, if the chin moves out and the head is extended, the rest of the body will move towards a supine recumbent position.

The application of Halliwick in the presence of balance deficits has prompted the integration of an activity, which I call sequential balance. This particular activity is of value in the treatment of patients who have lost function due to a stroke. Sequential balance (Figure 131) is practiced in shallow water. The therapist assumes the cube position (Figure 100) and the patient's hemiplegic side is seated on the therapist's opposite thigh (e.g., right hemiplegia on the left thigh). The therapist then proceeds to support the hemiplegic foot by placing his free foot over the patient's affected foot. The hemiplegic arm is at 90° flexion with the elbow extended in front of him. The patient's hand is held at the wrist by the therapist. The objective of this sequential balance activity is to gradually wean the patient off the support provided by the therapist as he acquires more balance, trunk control, and postural tone. The gradual wean implies removing first the foot, then the thigh, next the wrist support, and, finally, the patient maintains balance in the cube

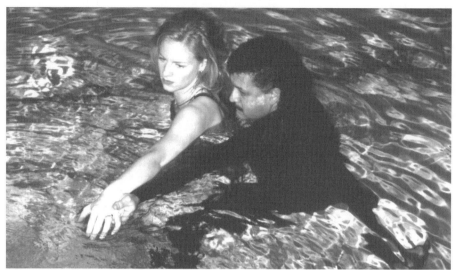

Figure 131: Sequential balance and weight shifting activities.

position on his own. Besides improving static balance, this activity additionally fosters weight bearing and weight-shifting.

Once a patient has achieved a certain level of motor control and postural tone, the kangaroo jumps may be integrated to improve dynamic balance and strengthen trunk control. The jump, which is a phase IV activity, involves marked flexion of the hip and knee with ankle dorsiflexion and some degree of hip abduction and external rotation (Figure 132). Patients with significant

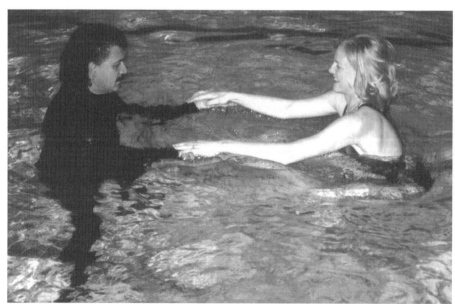

Figure 132: The kangaroo jumps.

balance deficits will not be able to perform this activity. They will have a tendency to lose their dynamic balance.

For patients exhibiting ataxia with some degree of extensor spasticity and a scissoring gait, the short-arm hold with integrated side-stepping or crab walk gait provides the means to inhibit tone and improve lower extremity coordination. If trunk control and balance are affected, lateral trunk movements can be gradually integrated, increasing the complexity of the activity.

Conclusion

Motor control of the trunk and extremities can be achieved through the practice of supine activities. Consider-ing that the Halliwick Method does not promote the use of floatation devices for its adapted activities, the patient assumes a specific position and alignment in the water by integrating breathing control and chin control techniques.

Although the Halliwick Method is widely practiced in pediatric patients exhibiting numerous neurological deficits, it has also been used success-fully in adult patients with strokes or other neurological problems. Patients with cerebellar dysfunction have been known to benefit from the application of Halliwick techniques.

CHAPTER 7

CLINICAL WASSERTANZEN

The term "Wassertanzen" literally translates into "Water Dancing." This aquatic bodywork approach was originally created by Arjana Brunschwiler and Aman Schröter in Belgium. It is a structured sequence of graceful movements with an emphasis on inducing relaxation, improving respiratory dynamics, decreasing tension, and increasing the mobility of the spine and weight-bearing joints.

Wassertanzen is an approach that integrates in an innovative way many of the flows and movements used in Watsu® with one unique difference, the patient experiences these sequences while submerged underwater for limited intervals of time. The movement sequences that are characteristic of Wassertanzen begin at water surface level and progress to more complex patterns that take the patient through a passive underwater experience. The practitioner is the active participant. Therefore, this individual must possess technical skill in the application of these sequential patterns of movement. The patient is the passive participant and, as such, must concentrate on relaxing, on how the relaxation process will affect his breathing cycle both at water surface level and on submersion, and on allowing himself to fully submit to and enjoy the experience.

In this chapter, I will discuss the potential benefits of Wassertanzen in an effort to establish its clinical relevance, leading to the development of my theories, which are based on observed respiratory and musculoskeletal physiology. Finally, concurrent with my identification of clinicopathologic correlations, I will present the clinical protocol that I developed and implemented in three phases, based on my analysis of this intervention.

Theories of Wassertanzen

In order to establish the clinical value of this approach based on my speculative theories, it is essential to seek for strong anatomical and musculoskeletal roots.

The first theory revolves around the influence of the central nervous system in respiratory function. Involuntary respiratory activity is controlled by the reticular formation located in the pons and the medulla oblongata (Figure 133). The pons lies anterior to the cerebellum and superior to the medulla oblongata. The medulla oblongata is a pyramidally shaped portion of the brain stem located between the spinal cord and the pons. These areas are, henceforth, known as the pontine-medullary center, or most commonly referred to as the respiratory centers. Conversely, voluntary respiratory activity such as the Valsalva maneuver, which is a breath-holding action, is controlled by the motor cortex. In my first theory, I maintain that *during a Wassertanzen session both the pontine-medullary center and the motor cortex are jointly recruited to contribute their integrated control and derive the ultimate benefits.* Therefore, the neurophysiological control of respiration is the foundation for

my first theory.

Furthermore, the pons and the medulla contain two secondary centers, which share in the control of respiration. These are the pneumotaxic center and the apneustic center (Figure 134). The pneumotaxic center is responsible for maintaining normal or adequate respiratory dynamics through facilitation of alternate inspiratory and expiratory activity. I call it the respiratory pacemaker. On the other hand, the apneustic center is not constantly active but will pick up activity when the pneumotaxic center slows down for some reason. When this happens, the pneumotaxic center is suddenly reactivated, inhibiting the apneustic center and resuming the normal respiratory pattern. On occasion we might find ourselves suddenly taking a deep sigh and then resuming our normal pattern of breathing. This is explained as a sudden activation of the apneustic center for a brief time.

Due to the impact that Wassertanzen has on the breathing cycle secondary to the repetitive facilitation of inspiratory function, I formulated my second theory in which I maintain that *activity of the apneustic center is strengthened during and after a*

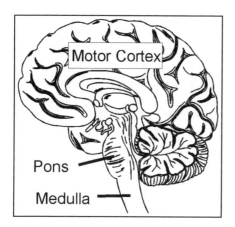

Figure 133: The brain showing the motor cortex, pons, and medulla oblongata.

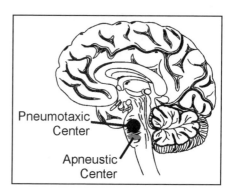

Figure 134: The pnemotaxic and apneustic centers of the pons.

Wassertanzen session. This is not meant to imply that the pneumotaxic center will become inactive, but rather that both centers are jointly sharing in a function that is primarily controlled by the pneumotaxic center. In other words, the apneustic center will function in the same capacity and at the same level as the respiratory pacemaker. This might account for such observed clinical signs and findings as:

1. a slower respiratory rate
2. an increase in the frequency of and tolerance to submersions
3. an increase in the frequency of involuntary deep inspiratory sighs experienced by the patients, which might last for several hours to several days following a Wassertanzen session.

The first two clinical objectives of Wassertanzen are directed towards improving the dynamics of respiration. One of these is the re-education of lung capacities and lung volumes with emphasis on expiratory reserve volume. Inspiratory capacity is defined as the amount of air that can be inspired at resting expiratory level. Inspiratory reserve volume is the amount of air that can be further inhaled at the end of a normal inspiration. Conversely, expiratory reserve volume is the amount of air that remains in the lungs and can be further exhaled after a normal expiration. With these three definitions in mind, I maintain that Wassertanzen will consequently have a positive effect on tidal volume and vital capacity. Tidal volume is defined as the amount of air that can be inhaled and exhaled in one breath. We refer to the amount of air that is exhaled after a maximal inspiration as vital capacity.

Another significant clinical objective of Wassertanzen is the neuromuscular re-education of the essential breathing patterns of respiration. There are two: diaphragmatic breathing and costolateral breathing (also called bibasilar excursions). Both patterns focus on strengthening the primary respiratory musculature, the diaphragm and intercostal muscles. This is an important consideration particularly for individuals who rely regularly on utilizing the accessory respiratory muscles due to weakness of the primary musculature. Optimizing the function of these muscles is of particular importance because it will subsequently reflect in normal closed chain thoracic kinematics and arthrokinematic activity.

Musculoskeletal re-education also figures among the clinical goals and objectives of Wassertanzen. When this is our main focus, the central goals are to improve optimal muscle strength, kinesthesia, and proprioception while at the same time inhibiting involuntary tension. Consequently, our attention should be focused on the sensory-motor receptors that contribute to an increase in muscle fiber contraction and to kinesthetic as well as proprioceptive awareness.

Two of the organelles that regulate muscle fiber activity are the muscle spindle and the Golgi tendon organ (GTO). The various movements and characteristic sequences of Wassertanzen produce a stretch on the primary and secondary intrafusal stretch receptors of the muscle spindle (Figure 135). These are usually referred to as type Ia and II fibers. A stretch of the muscle spindle will excite the extrafusal alpha motor neuron that will consequently activate the GTO causing inhibition of the antagonist. This will result in a stronger concentric contraction of the agonist through the excitation of motor units within the same muscle. This is a summarized interpretation of the applied principle of the stretch reflex.

Meanwhile, the alpha motor neurons or type I fibers act to influence proprioception and kinesthesia. Therefore, these receptors will provide sensory input on joint position and joint movement in space, which will ultimately affect movement direction, amplitude, speed, and relative tension.

There is a correlation between stretch reflex facilitation and the pontine-medullary function that has been linked with strengthening of the apneustic center. Improvement in the contractility of muscle fibers through stretch reflex facilitation will result in increased costolateral expansion, diaphragmatic function, and overall improved biomechanics of the thorax. Likewise, improvement in pulmonary ventilation and perfusion capabilities through stimulation of the respiratory centers and the key neuroanatomical structures will contribute to optimal respiratory dynamics.

Considering that stimulation and facilitation of internal and external respiratory dynamics occurs during Wassertanzen, I formulated my third theory. I maintain that *when diffusion takes place during a Wassertanzen session, the central and peripheral chemoreceptors become hypersensi-*

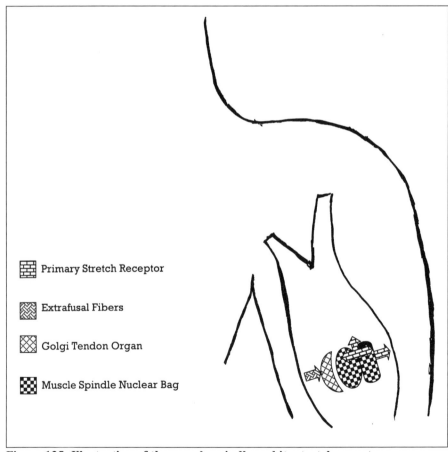

Figure 135: Illustration of the muscle spindle and its stretch receptors.

Legend:
- Primary Stretch Receptor
- Extrafusal Fibers
- Golgi Tendon Organ
- Muscle Spindle Nuclear Bag

tized. The result is a potential improvement in pulmonary compliance or the ease with which the lungs inflate and deflate, describing their recoil properties. Improving volumes and capacities will also improve the ventilation, perfusion, and diffusion capabilities of the lungs. If diffusion properties are enhanced, the pO_2 will, at the very least, be maintained at constant levels. The pO_2 represents the partial arterial pressure of oxygen diffused in plasma and is the product of the diffusion of oxygen at a pressure gradient through the alveolar-capillary membrane. Furthermore, as the airway becomes more pliable, transmural airway resistance will decrease.

The third clinical objective addresses the attainment of an optimal state of relaxation. All other objectives discussed are dependent on this one in order to derive the maximum benefits. When deep levels of relaxation are reached, the levels of consciousness may be altered. Concentrating on the breathing pattern for an extended period of time leads to a meditative state. As this meditative state is maintained, it leads an even higher state of consciousness. When a higher state of consciousness is reached and maintained for a period of time, a maximal state of consciousness is attained. Consequently, the attainment of optimal relaxation, which is essential in Wassertanzen, involves a progressive sequence of experiences that incorporate mind, body, and spirit.

The theories of relaxation in both Wassertanzen and Watsu® might be rooted in applied concepts of Yoga. According to these, the breathing cycle involves life energy, which is called Prana. Concentrating on our breathing dynamics leads to control of our life energy. This is referred to as Yama. As

we synchronize our breath with the applied movement sequences that are characteristic of Wassertanzen, we will ultimately expand our Prana. It is only when we expand our Prana that we will attain that higher state of consciousness that is our goal.

Based on a research study in fibromyalgia that I conducted, a final clinical objective that strengthens the clinical value of this aquatic therapy intervention is the inhibition of nociceptor activity. Nociceptors are those receptors responsible for producing pain. When nociceptor activity is inhibited, pain decreases. Two factors might contribute to this. First, the passive nature of the maneuvers and applied integrated release techniques lead to a potential resolution of muscle spasms and release of tight soft and myofascial tissue. The second factor is linked to the attained levels of relaxation.

Three Phases of Breathing Control

In order to properly retrain the primary respiratory musculature, the patient must learn to control his breathing both at water surface level and during submersions. In my analysis of the clinical relevance and physiologic basis of Wassertanzen, I describe a gradual process of breathing control that is accomplished in three phases:

Phase I – Breathing Control in the Upright Position

This technique uses hydrostatic pressure to offer resistance to the diaphragm and intercostal muscles. Normal breathing dynamics and exercises are practiced while sitting on a bench in the shallow area of the pool or standing in the cube position. The latter will also allow the therapist to work on postural alignment (Figure 136). The patient breathes in through the nose and out through the mouth. The water breath dance practiced in Watsu® is a typical activity integrated into this phase. Training the patient to master the essential breathing patterns is a fundamental aspect of this early phase of breathing control. While concentrating on diaphragmatic breathing, the patient should observe the increased abdominal pressure that is created when the diaphragmatic dome descends upon contraction. Lateral costal and basal excursions are another important consideration. When practicing these, hand placement should be emphasized in order to create awareness of thoracic kinematics and the bucket-handle movement of the ribs. Furthermore, attention should be paid to the concentric activity of the internal and external intercostal muscles.

Phase II – Breathing Control in the Supine Position

As the patient continues his practice of integrated diaphragmatic and costolateral breathing and as he enters into a state of relaxation, the practitioner cradles the patient in the supine position at water surface level (Figure 137). After performing a series of wavelike maneuvers with the objective of inducing relaxation and releasing tight soft and myofascial tissue, the therapist applies a nose clip to the patient (Figure 138). The pattern of breathing will now change to a mouth-breathing pattern. Towards the end of phase II, the patient will be briefly submerged for a few seconds. It is important to inform the patient about the transition to submersions once the patient assumes the supine position or during the orientation session. Just as important is informing the patient that prior to a submersion a sign will be given such as a double tap on any part of the body (back or extremities) or a double muscle squeeze. This sign will be given on exhalation before a

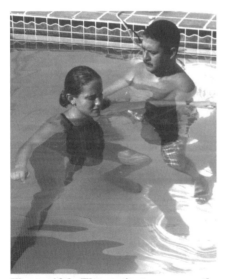

Figure 136: The patient assumes the cube position while the therapist examines postural alignment.

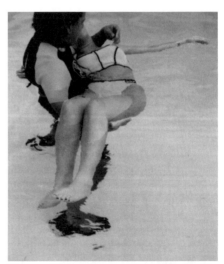

Figure 137: The head cradle in the supine position.

submersion event and will indicate that the patient will be submerged under water during the following exhalation. When this happens, the patient will exhale in small increments being careful not to fully exhale the air all at once. At first, submersions should not exceed three to five seconds.

Phase III – Breathing Control in Submersions

The progression of breathing control continues as the patient becomes more proficient in mastering his breath while submerged. Once proficiency is achieved, tolerance is also achieved and the time limits for submersion will gradually increase. When the patient is brought back to water surface level, it is important for the practitioner to observe and examine the patient's reaction and breathing pattern because this will serve as an indicator of the patient's level of tolerance to submersions. Even at optimal proficiency in this third phase, submersion time should be closely monitored each time. The therapist must be extremely attentive and watch for possible signs from the patient indicating his need to come back to the surface for air.

Clinical Wassertanzen

Clinical Wassertanzen is a structured protocol I designed and developed that is based on the three phases of breathing control that are discussed earlier in this chapter. I chose selected Brunschwiler and Schröter movement sequences. After a comprehensive analysis of this aquatic bodywork approach, in an effort to establish clinical value, I changed the original terminology used to designate the movement sequences. A more descriptive arthrokinematic terminology is used in this protocol with relevance to the anatomical and kinesiological effects on joints, muscles, ligaments, and myofascia.

Clinical Objectives

Three groups of clinical objectives have been identified based on the origi-

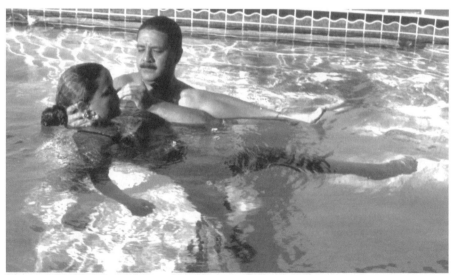

Figure 138: The therapist applies the nose clip to the patient.

nal theory. The cardiopulmonary objectives have been discussed earlier in this text. In summary, they address the following:

1. improvement in tidal volume and vital capacity
2. improvement in expiratory reserve volume
3. improvement in total lung capacity
4. strengthening of the primary respiratory musculature
5. improvement in cardiopulmonary endurance
6. improvement in thoracic kinematics
7. improvement in the ventilation, perfusion and diffusion capabilities of the lungs.

The second group of objectives impact soft tissue, connective tissue, and articular structures. These musculoskeletal objectives include:

1. improvement in muscle strength
2. improvement in range of motion
3. improvement in joint flexibility and mobility
4. reduction in spasmodic activity
5. improvement in the elasticity and plasticity of connective tissue
6. enhancement in the ability to achieve optimal relaxation
7. reduction of pain
8. improvement in proprioceptive and kinesthetic awareness.

The third clinical objective focuses on the benefits derived by the patient once he has attained optimal levels of relaxation. I have proven through a research study conducted on a patient with fibromyalgia that the achievement of optimal levels of relaxation will lead to an improvement in non-REM sleep patterns.

Applied Passive Maneuvers

The protocol described later in the chapter identifies four types of applied passive maneuvers:

1. The *trunk and spine* maneuvers are those that have a direct impact on the cervical, thoracic, and lumbar spines as well as on the sacroiliac joint. Integrated techniques such as distraction or passive movement of a joint through the full or partial range figure in this type of maneuver. A typical example is the prone snaking maneuver.

2. The maneuvers of the *pelvic belt musculature* (originally referred to as the lower extremity aikido sequences) promote lumbar pelvic rhythm with an emphasis on range of motion of the hip joint and soft-tissue stretch to the constituents of the pelvic belt, namely the hip flexors, extensors, and external rotators.

3. The third type consists of the *lower extremity* maneuvers. Some specific integrated techniques, such as the recovery technique from the prone snaking maneuvers, are featured in this type because they involve passive ranges of two major lower extremity joints. Likewise, portions of the aikido sequences might be considered within the realm of lower extremity maneuvers. The lumbosacral stabilization maneuver, which is the tenth step of Phase III, is a classic example because of its impact on the acetabulofemoral, tibiofemoral, and tibiotalar joints through integrated joint approximation techniques and anteroposterior glides.

4. The last type of applied passive maneuvers is characterized by those that have a direct effect on

the shoulder joint or the shoulder girdle. These are the *upper extremity* maneuvers. The scapulohumeral distraction maneuver and the scapulothoracic mobilization maneuver featured in Phase III Steps 7 and 8 are examples of this group. These maneuvers also have an indirect impact on the pectoral girdle as well as distally on the elbow and wrist joints.

Integrated Techniques

Within each applied passive maneuver, there are a series of integrated manual techniques implemented to enhance or produce specific effects as a means towards goal attainment:
1. *Passive range of motion* is applied to improve concave-convex joint surface relationships. Passive joint range occurs in all three cardinal planes.
2. *Passive manual stretches* are applied to muscles and ligaments in selected maneuvers. These might be performed statically in a single specific technique or dynamically in combination with a movement sequence.

3. Applied *myofascial and soft tissue releases* are integrated throughout the protocol. Phase II focuses on the integrated application of these techniques. Of particular importance, trigger point releases to the soft tissue are effective in the resolution of spasmodic activity.
4. *Applied joint distraction and approximation techniques* are specifically integrated in upper and lower extremity maneuvers when the clinical objective is to increase range of motion, decrease pain, and improve kinesthetic awareness.
5. Finally, *joint mobilization techniques* are featured as a highlight to passive distraction maneuvers or soft tissue releases.

Considerations

The Clinical Wassertanzen Protocol should be modified and adapted to each type of patient considering the identified clinical problems as well as related indications or contraindications. For instance, the anteroposterior glides, which characterize the acetabulofemoral component of Step 10 in Phase III, are contraindicated in patients with

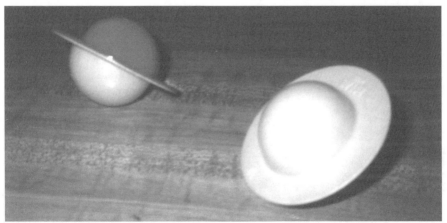

Figure 139: The spherical Saturn flip eggs used in the first Phase I activity.

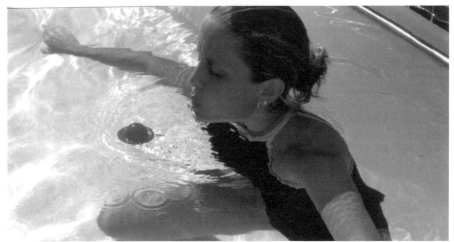

Figure 140: Upon instruction by the therapist, the patient practices tidal volume and vital capacity retraining using the Saturn flip egg.

a hip arthroplasty in order to avoid the risk of a dislocation of the prosthetic joint.

Clinical Wassertanzen Protocol

Phase I: Breathing Control in the Upright Position

Exercise 1: Tidal Volume and Vital Capacity Retraining

This exercise requires the use of the Saturn flip eggs, which are also used in selected Halliwick breathing activities. These are plastic spherical objects with a flat ring in the center around its circumference that allows them to float in the water (Figure 139). The patient is instructed to take a deep inspiration and fully exhale on the surface of the water, flipping the objects over repeatedly until the expiration phase ends (Figure 140). It is important to count the number of flips the patient completes on full expiratory effort. This is followed by a rest interval and then the exercise is repeated.

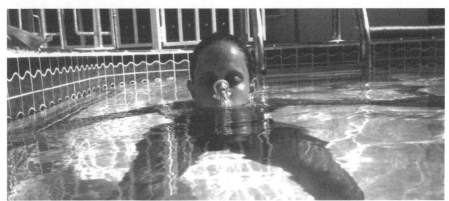

Figure 141: The patient practices post-expiratory endurance stage 1.

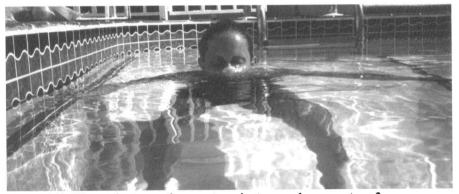

Figure 142: The patient practices post-expiratory endurance stage 2.

Exercise 2: Post Expiratory Endurance

This exercise is completed in three stages. A nose clip is required but goggles might be worn at the patient's or therapist's discretion.

Stage 1

The patient assumes the cube position while holding a handrail. After taking a deep breath, the patient begins a partial submersion. The water level should be slightly above the upper lip (Figure 141). Once partially submerged, the patient slowly exhales fully, forming bubbles on the surface of the water. After the full expiratory effort has been completed, the patient maintains this position for as long as he can tolerate it. At this point, the therapist records the time from the end of the expiratory phase to the time when the patient needs to rise up for air again. When the patient feels comfortable with this activity and has progressed in endurance to partial submersions, he can move on to stage 2.

Stage 2

The patient repeats the same submersion exercise described in stage 1 but this time the partial submersion occurs to the level of the roof of the nose (Figure 142). The same procedure is followed. The therapist times the post-expiratory endurance period.

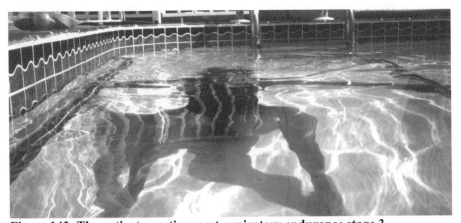

Figure 143: The patient practices post-expiratory endurance stage 3.

Stage 3

The same exercise described in stage 2 is repeated. This time there will be a full submersion. The patient squats down, so that his head is fully submersed under the water (Figure 143). In order to ensure that the patient is comfortable under the water, it is advisable for the patient to maintain a reasonable amount of hip abduction and external rotation with hip flexion. However, when this position is contraindicated, the patient can kneel and then sit on the legs or maintain the hips adducted. The therapist can also assist the patient by passively leaning him forward or backwards if difficulty with the self-submersion exercise is experienced. Once again, the therapist times post-expiratory endurance.

Exercise 3: The Water Breath Dance

This exercise has been adapted and carried over to this protocol from the common practice of Watsu® and the original sequential program of Wasser-tanzen. The patient assumes the cube position and begins the process of relaxation by gently inhaling and exhaling through normal breathing dynamics, that is, in through the nose and out through the mouth (Figure 144). He should become aware of the buoyancy effects of this exercise as his body rises when he inhales and sinks when he exhales. The patient should find a comfortable place in the pool, preferably against the wall because this is the spot the patient will return to at the end of the session.

This exercise marks the transition into Phase II. When the patient feels that the relaxation process has begun, the therapist walks towards the right side of the patient and places the cubital fossa of his left arm against the extensor surface of the patient's neck, cradling the head. The patient is then instructed to lean back and float in the supine position. The right arm of the therapist now holds the patient's knees at the popliteal surface.

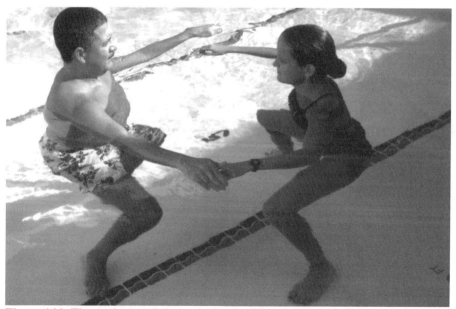

Figure 144: The patient and therapist begin the water breath dance.

Phase II: Breathing Control in the Supine Position

This phase consists of five steps that integrate a series of manual techniques introduced earlier in this chapter.

Step 1: Applied lateral sacral glides

With the patient in the supine position cradled by the therapist, the practitioner now placed his left hand with the knuckles facing upwards (Figure 145 and Figure 146) against the median crest of the sacrum and begins to move the sacrum from side to side.

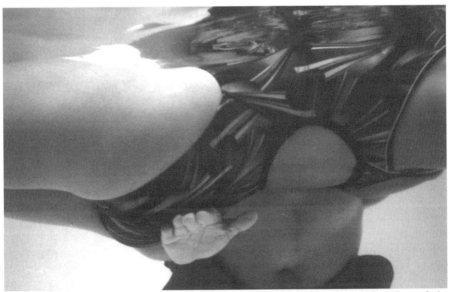

Figure 145: Underwater view of the hand placement for the application of the lateral sacral glides. Moving from side...

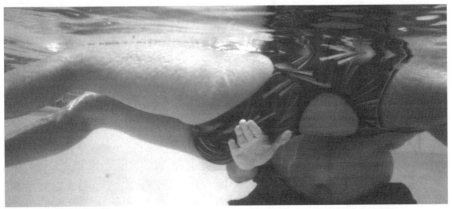

Figure 146: ...to side.

Step 2: Applied soft tissue and myofascial releases (STR and MFR)

This maneuver focuses primarily on the application of manual stretches. The first integrated technique is a passive stretch to the unilateral lumbodorsal fascia and quadratus lumborum on the near side (Figure 147). Secondly, a contralateral and unilateral stretch to the oblique muscles of the abdomen and to the intercostal muscles is applied (Figure 148). Paraspinal soft tissue release with trigger point applications is the third technique. The therapist uses the heel and fingertips of the four medial digits of his hand to apply pressure to the intrinsic paraspinal muscles as he "walks" up the spine from the sacrum to the midscapular region (Figure 149 and Figure 150).

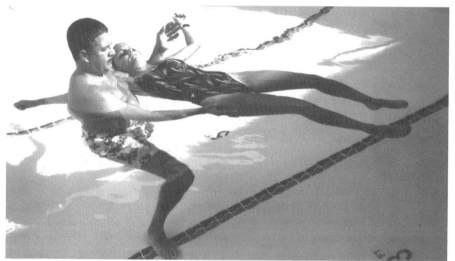

Figure 147: Unilateral passive stretches to the ipsilateral lumbodorsal fascia and quadratus lumborum muscle.

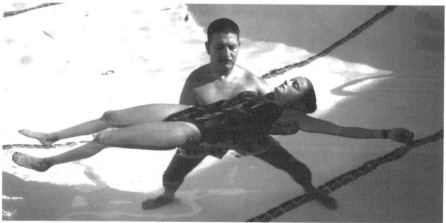

Figure 148: Unilateral passive stretches to the contralateral obliques and intercostal muscles.

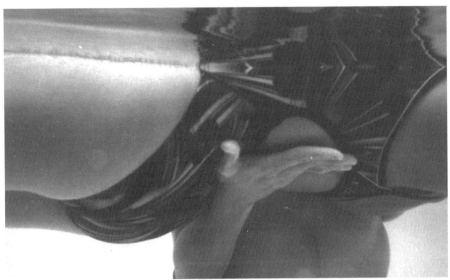

Figure 149: Underwater view demonstrating the application of the paraspinal releases. Moving...

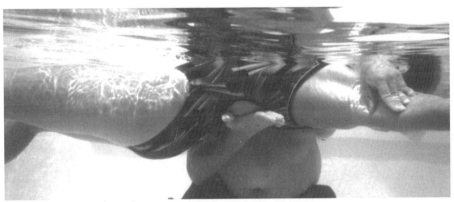

Figure 150: ...up the spine.

The paraspinal muscles affected are the longissimus, spinalis, multifidi, and rotatores.

Step 3: Trigger Point Release (TPR)

This technique consists of the application of pressure on pain-sensitive areas known as trigger points. The main cause of pain is increased spasmodic activity. In the area of the trigger point, the patient might exhibit varying grades of spasmodic activity ranging from grades 1 to 4 as described in the Spas-

modic Activity Grading Scale in Chapter 2. In addition to the trigger point release technique, this maneuver allows the practitioner to apply pétrissage and effleurage to the cervical extensors and scapular muscles in an effort to further release tight soft and myofascial tissue.

The therapist holds the back of the patient's knees and brings the patient into a sitting position (Figure 151). Once the patient is held in a sitting

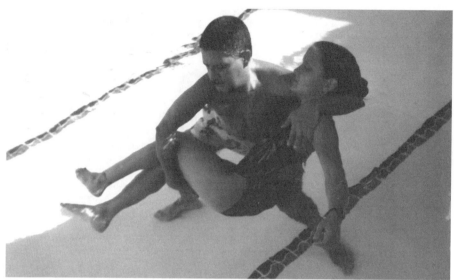

Figure 151: Bringing the patient to a sitting position in preparation for the application of trigger point releases.

position, the therapist clamps his knees on the patient's knees to secure him in this position. The patient's head is passively moved to rest on the therapist's left arm. This position will allow the therapist to work on the application of trigger point releases and soft tissue

massage to the right cervical and scapular area.

Step 4: Cervical Spine Distraction

Once the therapist has unilaterally worked on trigger point releases, he will hold the patient's head with both

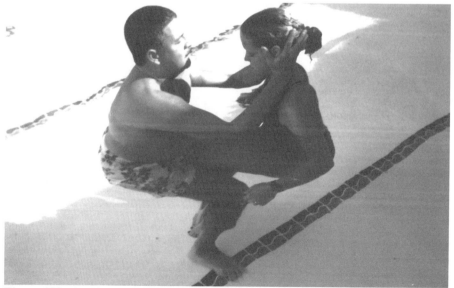

Figure 152: Application of the cervical distraction maneuver.

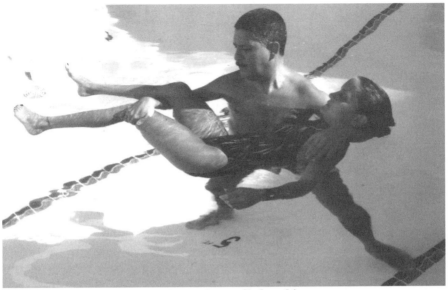

Figure 153: The therapist performs the cradled rocking maneuver.

hands, placing it in axial extension, and proceed with a distraction maneuver of the cervical spine while gently swinging the body in a pendulum action (Figure 152). Once the distraction maneuver is completed, the therapist performs a "head turn." This movement turns the patient onto the opposite side where the therapist can repeat Steps 2 and 3.

Step 5: Cradled Rocking
    A head turn is performed to bring the therapist back to the patient's right

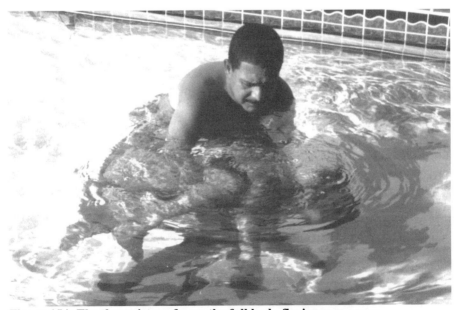

Figure 154: The therapist performs the full body flexion maneuver.

side. The therapist should monitor the patient's breathing pattern and coordinate his breathing with the rocking movements. The patient's head is cradled during the rocking maneuver while the therapist's right arm is threaded under the back of the patient's right knee with the hand grasping his left knee (Figure 153). Short interval submersions lasting between three and five seconds begin during this maneuver. This is the transition maneuver to Phase III.

The patient's position with the therapist's arm threaded through the knee allows the therapist to bring the patient momentarily into a sitting position so that the nose clip can be applied (Figure 138).

Phase III: Breathing Control in Submersion

This phase has twelve steps that combine all of the integrated techniques described previously within a series of passive maneuvers.

Step 1: Passive full body flexion

In this maneuver, the patient is brought to a side-lying fetal position. The combination of movements consists of bilateral hip and knee flexion with spine flexion on all regions, thereby facilitating lumbar pelvic rhythm (Figure 154). During the full body flexion maneuver, the patient is released from the cradled position so that one the therapist's hands is placed on the patient's right shoulder while the other is flexing the hips and knees. This is followed by the recovery position of full body extension. The therapist's hand placement in recovery is always at the occiput and popliteal surface of the knees (Figure 155).

Step 2: Passive maneuver of the pelvic belt musculature with proximal hold

After the submersion signal is given, the therapist wraps his right arm around the patient's right thigh. The practitioner proceeds to passively move the hip into flexion by exerting gentle pressure on the anterior superior iliac spine (Figure 156) with alternate hip hyperextension where the pressure is

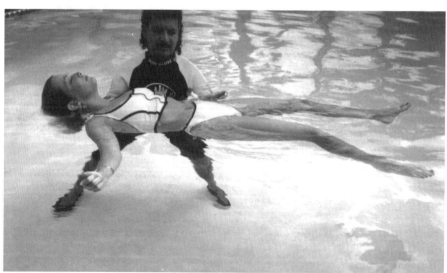

Figure 155: The standard recovery position.

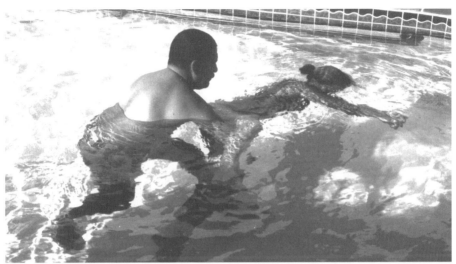

Figure 156: The first component of the pelvic belt passive maneuver with proximal hold.

exerted on the ischial tuberosity (Figure 157). The maneuver is performed in a gentle sweeping sequence of movements. The proximal-hold passive technique will produce an alternate, unilateral stretch on soft tissues and connective tissues. The soft tissues affected during the flexion-extension component of the maneuver are the iliopsoas and gluteus maximus muscles. Connective tissue structures such as the Y ligament of Bigelow anteriorly and the sacrotuberous, sacrospinous, and sacroiliac ligaments posteriorly are also stretched. Likewise, the passive acetabulofemoral and sacroiliac range of motion that occurs during this maneuver will impact joint arthrokinematics. The hip will flex past 90° with an estimated 45° of hyperextension taking place during the second component of the maneuver.

Step 3: Passive maneuver of the pelvic belt musculature with distal hold

The same technique discussed in Step 2 is applied in this maneuver. The

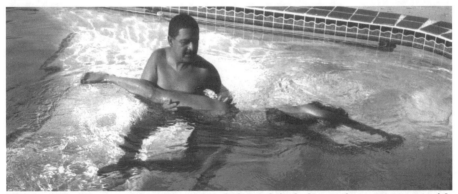

Figure 157: The second component of the pelvic belt passive maneuver with proximal hold.

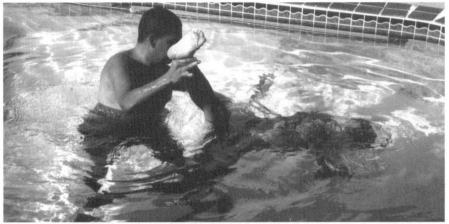

Figure 158: Hand placement at the ankle joint in preparation for the application of the pelvic belt passive maneuver with distal hold.

only difference is the distal hold at the right talocrural joint (Figure 158). If at all possible, the knee is maintained in extension. However, some limited flexion might be permitted if it cannot be avoided. This maneuver has an impact on the same soft and connective tissue structures identified in Step 2. However, due to the distal hold technique, two additional soft tissue struc-

tures, the sartorius and the rectus femoris muscles, are affected because of their proximal origin in the os coxae. The estimated range of motion in hip flexion and hyperextension remains as described in Step 2.

In order to turn the patient to the opposite side and perform the same maneuvers described in Steps 2 and 3, the therapist has the option of per-

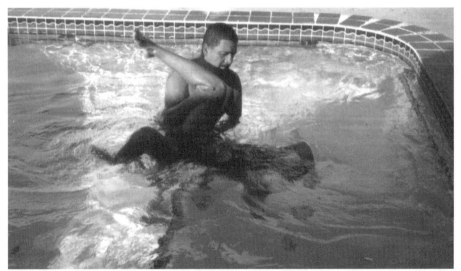

Figure 159: The semicircular somersault as an optional technique to turn the patient to the opposite side.

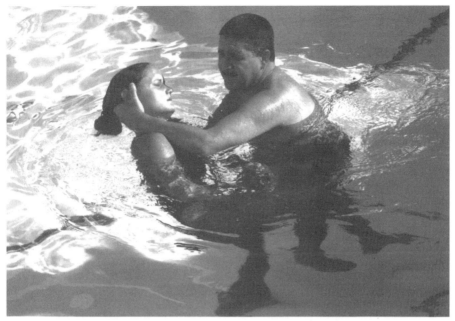

Figure 160: The head turn as an optional technique to switch the patient to the opposite side.

forming a semicircular somersault (Figure 159).

The semicircular somersault flips the patient around to the prone position after which the patient is turned around to the other side at the thighs. Another option is to perform a simple head turn as described in Phase II (Figure 160).

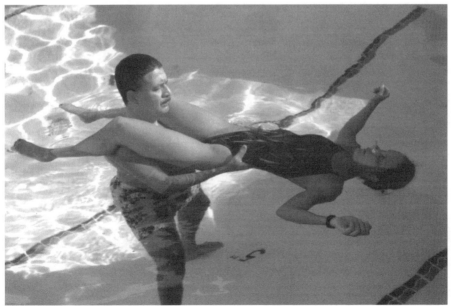

Figure 161: Position of the patient in preparation for the application of the passive pelvic and spine rotations.

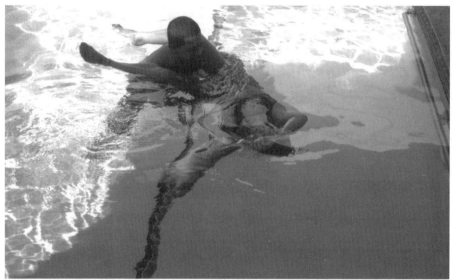

Figure 162: The therapist performs the pelvic and spine rotations in submersion applying a figure of eight pattern.

The same techniques can be repeated whenever a maneuver is performed unilaterally to allow the practitioner to complete the maneuver on the opposite side.

Step 4: Passive pelvic and spine rotations

During the first component of Step 4, the patient's left leg is placed to rest

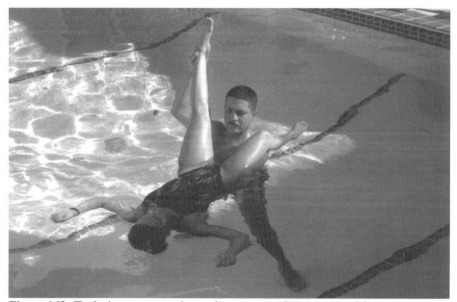

Figure 163: Technique to turn the patient over to the prone position.

on the therapist's right shoulder. Gently, the other leg is placed at the left shoulder allowing the therapist to hold the patient's trunk (Figure 161). After the signal, the therapist holds both hips at the iliac crests and begins to partially rotate the innominate bones around a transverse axis in a figure of eight pattern (Figure 162). When one innominate bone is rotated downward, the other one is rotated upward. This maneuver releases the sacroiliac joint.

Step 5: Prone spine snaking maneuver

This maneuver facilitates passive, alternate flexion and extension movements of all the vertebral regions. Although the direct impact of the passive movements is strongest at the zygapophyseal joints of the vertebrae, it is also felt distally at the glenohumeral, acetabulofemoral, tibiofemoral, and tibiotalar joints in succession.

The therapist reaches for the patient's left ankle with his right hand, lifts the leg up, and turns the patient over to the prone position (Figure 163). Once the patient is in the prone position, the therapist grabs both ankles, locking them together as both index fingers and thumbs touch. With swift movements up and down, the therapist will create an undulating wavelike motion of the patient's body (Figure 164).

The most difficult part of this maneuver is the recovery technique. It consists of bilaterally abducting the patient's lower extremities and sending them towards each side of the therapist allowing the practitioner to simultaneously catch the patient at the popliteal surfaces of both knees (Figure 165). As the patient is brought to a sitting position, his head will rest on the therapist's right shoulder, and his hips and knees will be maximally flexed. In this recovery position, the practitioner can now perform alternate passive short-arc hip and knee flexion to the end range with adductor stretch.

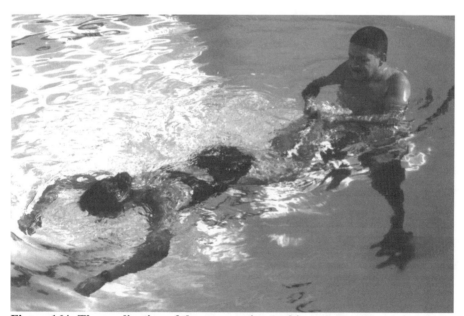

Figure 164: The application of the prone spine snaking maneuver.

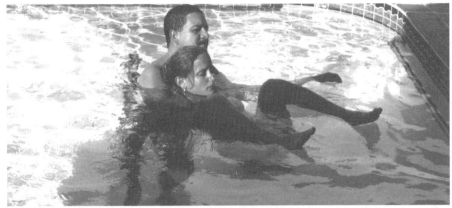

Figure 165: The recovery technique and position following the prone spine snaking maneuver.

Step 6: Passive thoracolumbar flexion and extension

The therapist sways forward gently dropping the patient once again in the prone position (Figure 166). Hand placement for this particular maneuver is at the thoracic spine over the spinous processes and at the lower third of the sternum and xiphoid process. The therapist applies alternate pressure on the thoracic spine and the sternum, which will be distally reflected on the glenohumeral and acetabulofemoral

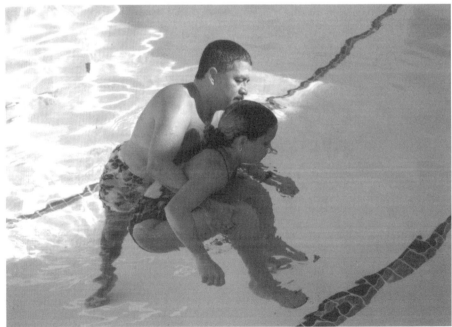

Figure 166: The technique to place the patient in the prone position in preparation for Step 6 of the Submersion Phase.

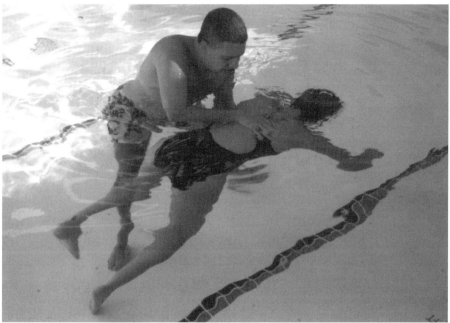

Figure 167: The application of alternate pressure in the thoracic spine and sternum in the prone position.

joints (Figure 167).

The patient is turned to the supine position and back to water surface level by a simple turn at his thighs.

Step 7: Scapulohumeral distraction

This applied passive maneuver concentrates exclusively on the upper extremities. The integrated distraction techniques will have a distal impact on the humeroulnar and radiocarpal joints. The passive movements that are performed within the maneuver are gentle rotations of the glenohumeral joint bringing the patient under the water and

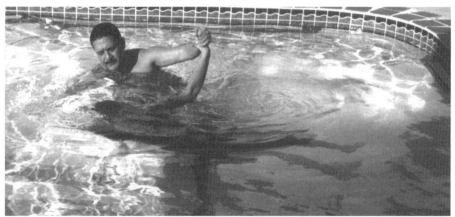

Figure 168: The therapist prepares to perform the scapulohumeral distraction maneuver.

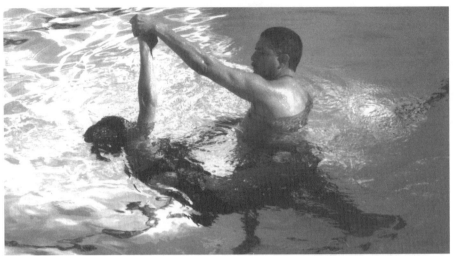

Figure 169: The application of alternate scapulohumeral distractions.

back to water surface level. The distraction technique is applied at the end of the sequence of passive movements and rotations.

The therapist will reach for the patient's left hand with his right hand locking the patient's thumb securely between his thumb and index finger (Figure 168). He then reaches for the right hand with his right hand applying the same locking technique of the thumb. Another option for hand placement is at the wrist joints. As the pa-

tient is submersed, the therapist begins to rotate the patient around swinging his arms and rotating him around an axis (Figure 169). It is important to maintain a secure grip on the patient's hands at all times.

A distraction of the patient's left shoulder in a 90° flexed position will permit cradling of the head or hand placement at the occiput bringing the patient back to the standard recovery position (Figure 170).

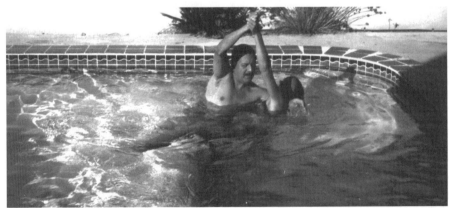

Figure 170: Return to the head cradle and standard recovery position following the scapulohumeral distraction maneuver.

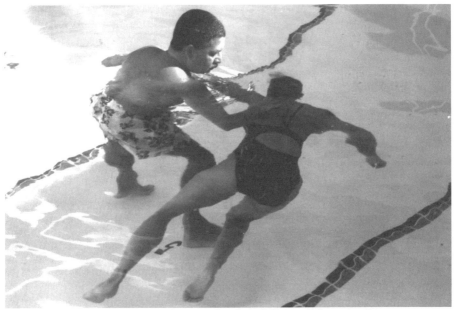

Figure 171: The therapist works on releasing tight scapular muscles.

Step 8: Scapulothoracic mobilization

This maneuver not only focuses on mobilization of the scapulothoracic joint but on soft tissue releases as well. The therapist reaches for the patient's left hand with his left hand and turns the patient to the prone position. While still holding the patient's hand, the therapist's other hand is free to work on the scapular muscles (Figure 171).

A gentle push near the scapulohumeral region will turn the patient around and back to the standard recovery position.

Step 9: Cervicothoracolumbar spine rotations

The therapist's right hand holds the patient at both ankles or the back of

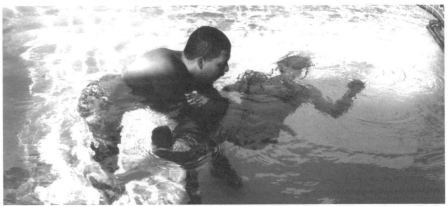

Figure 172: The therapist applies spine rotations at all levels in sweeping figure of eight movements.

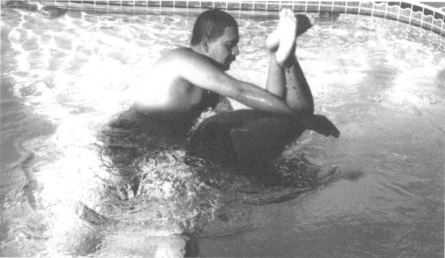

Figure 173: The transfer somersault flip is a technique to turn the patient to the opposite side.

both knees. The other hand rests on the lower abdomen gently flexing the hip and submersing the patient. The position of the therapist's left hand remains in contact with the patient while sweeping the patient side to side in rotational and figure of eight motions

(Figure 172).

The transfer somersault flip is the recovery technique for this maneuver if a change to the opposite side is considered. The turning of the patient begins at the legs with a flip to the prone position followed by a turn into the

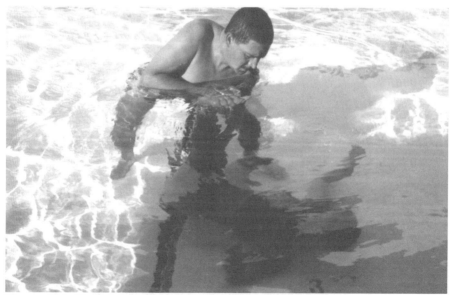

Figure 174: Technique and hand placement used for lumbosacral and pelvic stabilization in submersion.

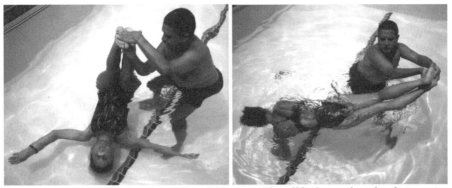

Figure 175: Hand placement and technique used to lift the patient back to water surface level in order to assume the standard recovery position.

supine position and back to water surface level (Figure 173).

Step 10: Lumbosacral and pelvic stabilization with integrated joint approximation and anteroposterior glides

Once again, hand placement is at the ankles. The knees are maintained extended and the patient is lowered until his back is resting comfortably on the bottom surface of the pool followed by stabilization of the hips and sacrum.

A 90° angle of bilateral hip flexion is maintained. One hand should secure knee extension while the other is moved up to the plantar surfaces of both feet (Figure 174). In this position, tibiofemoral joint approximation can be integrated. Another optional integrated technique consists of the application of gentle anteroposterior glides to the acetabulofemoral joint.

The hand that is placed at the anterior surface of the knees moves up to

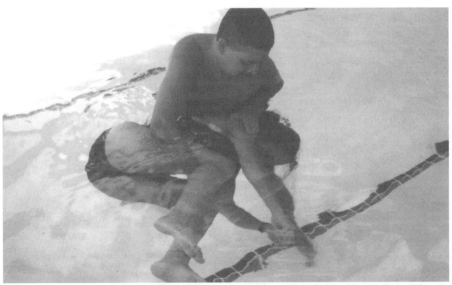

Figure 176: A partially sustained full body flexion maneuver where the patient's head rests on the therapist's thigh.

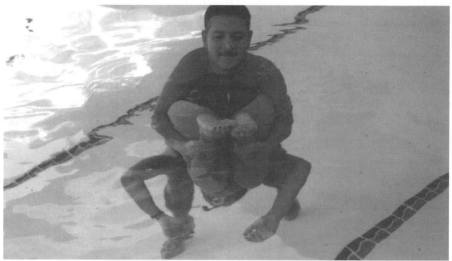

Figure 177: A partially sustained full body flexion maneuver with full inversion of the body in submersion where the patient's shoulders rest on the therapist's thighs.

the dorsum of the feet as the patient's legs are lifted and swung up and over bringing the patient back to the standard recovery position (Figure 175).

Step 11: Passive full body flexion

The passive full body flexion maneuver is repeated. At this point, the therapist might consider temporarily

resting the patient's head and neck on his left thigh (Figure 176), or the patient can be completely inverted with his head down and his shoulders resting between the therapist's thighs (Figure 177). The latter will allow the therapist to hold the patient at his knees with both arms, maximizing knee and hip flexion.

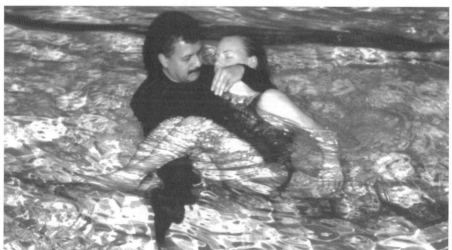

Figure 178: Bilateral repetitive hip flexion-extension pattern at water surface.

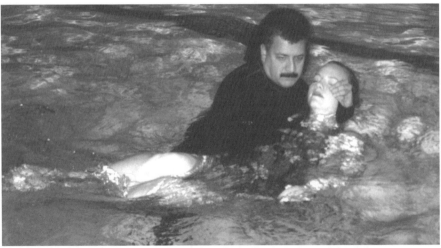

Figure 179: Bilateral repetitive rotational hip flexion-extension pattern.

Step 12: Watsu® sequence

Two Watsu® sequential movements will conclude the third phase of the protocol and ultimately the Clinical Wassertanzen session. These are the bilateral repetitive hip and knee flexion-extension pattern (Figure 178) and the bilateral repetitive hip rotation with integrated flexion-extension pattern (Figure 179).

The patient is slowly and gradually brought back to the starting point of the session and the original sitting position. Shoulders and knees are properly secured and aligned before the therapist distances himself from the patient. He then waits for a reaction from the patient.

Conclusion

In addition to its use as a wellness approach and in sports medicine, Wassertanzen has proven effective in providing symptomatic relief in patients with fibromyalgia. Patients who present with clinical evidence of widespread spasmodic activity, limited range of motion, tight myofascial tissue, disturbance of sleep patterns, and pain or tenderness have benefited from the application of the passive maneuvers and integrated manual techniques described in this protocol.

Considering the results of the pilot study discussed in Part III of this text, which shows the effects of Wassertanzen in relieving muscle spasms and pain and on improving sleep patterns, I now advocate using this technique on orthopedic conditions. Considering the theories and clinical objectives discussed in this chapter, Wassertanzen might also prove to be an effective aquatic therapy intervention in selected neurological and cardiopulmonary conditions. However, in these cases, the patient's diagnosis and clinical findings are a factor in the modification of the protocol to include those phases, techniques, or maneuvers that are best suited for each diagnosis with emphasis on indications and contraindications.

CHAPTER 8
CARDIAQUATICS

Cardiaquatics is a structured, four-level, multi-sequence protocol consisting of integrated phase IV cardiac rehabilitation and aquatic activities performed in a swimming pool. It fosters group exercises in a dynamic setting. Music can be used in selected levels as an incentive for the patient. The Cardiaquatics Protocol I designed and developed in 1996 was the result of my prior experience and work in the area of cardiopulmonary physical therapy.

The functional outcomes of the Cardiaquatics Protocol focus on two key clinical objectives:
1. To maintain a physiologic homeostasis through optimal cardiopulmonary fitness
2. To promote wellness.

Overview of Cardiac Rehabilitation

In order to understand the objective and structure of the Cardiaquatics protocol the reader must first have knowledge of cardiac rehabilitation, its phases, goals, guidelines, and physical activities.

Cardiac rehabilitation is the process of actively assisting a patient known to have cardiac problems to achieve and maintain an optimal state of health. It is divided into four phases that are designated by roman numerals. Phases I and II are considered inpatient phases, meaning that they are carried out while the patient is in the hospital. Phases III and IV are outpatient phases. In other words, they are administered after the patient has been discharge from the hospital.

Phase I

The goal of Phase I is to prevent the deconditioning effects resulting from the cardiac event or from the prolonged bed rest associated with the cardiac event. The clinical signs that are

149

associated with deconditioning include but are not limited to:

1. muscle weakness
2. tachycardia
3. thrombus formation
4. constipation
5. orthostatic hypotension
6. pulmonary congestion.

Phase I cardiac rehabilitation consists of a structured protocol, which features a program of physical activities along with ward or self-care activities that are supervised by a therapist who has experience in this area. The physical activities featured in phase I range from passive range of motion exercises to ambulating specified distances within the room or sitting for a determined period of time. One example of a popular phase I program used in a clinic setting is the Wenger's 14-Step Protocol (Table 2). Other, more complex protocols have been designed for a specific diagnostic group or for a specific type of clinic.

The contraindications for admitting a patient into phase I cardiac rehabilitation include evidence of complications such as congestive heart failure, uncontrolled ventricular arrhythmias, and/or unstable angina, which is also known as class IV angina pectoris or angina at rest.

The physical activities that form part of the phase I cardiac rehabilitation program are regulated by guidelines addressing:

1. the progression of activities through the program
2. the involvement of the patient as an active participant in the program
3. the patient's capabilities to perform the activity
4. rules for patient monitoring in order to determine progress or noncompliance.

Basic monitoring procedures consist of recording blood pressure and heart rate on a flow sheet in the patient's chart. Include a telemetry rhythm strip if the patient happens to be on telemetry or has a cardiac monitor in place. A patient may be placed on hold or discontinued altogether from cardiac rehabilitation if he experiences one or more of these contraindications:

1. angina within the past twenty-four hours
2. evidence of an irregular pulse
3. lightheadedness upon standing
4. nausea, vomiting, or diaphoresis
5. a resting high or low blood pressure based on the patient's medical history to date
6. a resting high or low heart rate based on the patient's medical history to date
7. dyspnea.

The progression of the patient through the phase I program will depend on the absence or evidence of established disproportionate responses to the physical activities. Established disproportionate responses may include:

1. an increase in systolic blood pressure of over twenty millimeters of mercury
2. a decrease in systolic blood pressure of over ten millimeters of mercury
3. evidence of arrhythmias
4. a heart rate exceeding 120 beats per minute
5. an ataxic gait.

Designed by Dr. Nanette Wenger, the Wenger's Protocol (Table 2) is the most frequently utilized phase I and II cardiac rehabilitation instrument. It consists of fourteen physical activity steps with integrated self-care activities. I consider steps 1 through 6 as the key physical activities in phase I.

Table 2: The Wenger's 14-Step Cardiac Rehabilitation Protocol.

Step	Physical Activity	Self-Care Activity
1 & 2	Passive ROM/ankle pumps	Bed rest; self-feeding
3	Active assistive ROM	Wash hand & face, shave, dangle legs, commode, bathe above waist, OOB to chair x2 for 30 min.
4	Active ROM	Change gown, OOB to chair x3 for 45 min.
5	Active ROM with min. resistance; ambulation to 25 ft. within room x2	Dressing, combing hair, bathroom privileges, sitting x2 up to 3 hours
6	Active ROM with min. resistance at bedside; ambulation to 50 ft. within room x2	Stand at sink to shave; sitting ad lib
7	Standing warm ups: arm/shoulder circles x5, stand on toes x10 plus ambulation to 100 ft. x2	
8	Warm ups: lateral trunk flexion x5 and trunk twists x5 plus ambulation to 200 ft. x2	
9	Warm ups: lateral trunk flexion w/1 lb. wt. x10, knee to chest x5, trunk twists x5 w/1 lb. wt. and knee bends x10 plus ambulation to 300 ft. x2	
10	Same as Step 9 plus ambulation to 400 ft. x2	
11	Same as Step 10 plus leg raises x5 and ambulation to 400 ft. x2	Shower privileges
12	Lateral trunk flexion w/2 lb. wt. x10, leg raises x10, trunk twists x10 w/2 lb. wt. stairs: 4 steps up/down in PT Clinic plus ambulation to 600 ft. x2	
13	Same as Step 12 plus full flight of stairs up/down and ambulation to 800 ft. x2	
14	Same as Step 12 plus touch toes from sitting x10, full stairs x2, and ambulation to 1000 ft. x2	

Characteristically, these activities begin with passive range of motion. This activity may start on the coronary care unit and end with ambulation within the room when the patient has been transferred to the recovery floor.

Phase II

As a continuation of phase I, phase II cardiac rehabilitation indicates that the patient is moving in the right direc-tion for successful recovery. Since steps 1 through 6 of the Wenger's Protocol have been identified as the phase I components, phase II will consist of steps 7 through 14. The physical activi-ties in the phase II protocol vary from ambulation outside the patient's room with progressively increasing distances to stair climbing.

The highlight of phase II cardiac rehabilitation is the integration of a program of patient and family educa-tion. Audiovisual aids are used in these inservices in order to enhance the presentation and the learning process. The educational inservices featured in phase two include the following:

1. physical activities and discharge teaching conducted by the therapist
2. risk-factor modification conducted by the nurse or nutritionist
3. medications and their effects conducted by the nurse or physician
4. dealing with heart attack symptoms conducted by the nurse or physician
5. the effects of smoking on coronary artery disease with emphasis on nicotine and carbon monoxide effects conducted by the therapist, nurse, or physician.

Discharge of the patient from the hospital marks the culmination of phase II cardiac rehabilitation.

Phase III

The goal of phase III cardiac rehabilitation is to assist the patient to return safely to his usual activities or to find acceptable substitutes for activities that are not appropriate. Therefore, the activities in phase III are designed to help the patient gradually regain strength and confidence.

The traditional exercise prescription is the daily walk. The physician and therapist will determine the intensity and distance, which will depend on the incidence of complications during the course of recovery and the extent of the cardiac event. When it is indicated upon the approval of the physician following a stress test, the patient might be referred to an outpatient therapy clinic to undergo a monitored exercise program. The structure of the outpatient phase III cardiac rehabilitation program consists of three segments:

1. the warm up segment, which features a program of low impact cardiac calisthenics performed to stimulate circulation and respiratory adjustments, to loosen joints and muscles, to reduce strain, and to increase muscle and body temperature
2. the training segment, which is the longest lasting, approximately twenty to thirty minutes and consisting of a progressive routine of walking to speed walking to jogging
3. the cool down segment, characterized by light activity such as breathing exercises or slow paced walking performed to avoid venous pooling in the lower extremities and the side effects resulting from venous stasis.

Phase IV

The objective of phase IV cardiac rehabilitation is to assist the patient to maintain an optimal physical state through a safe and structured advanced exercise-training program. Therefore, phase IV will focus on cardiovascular fitness. Phase IV programs can be supervised or unsupervised, and characteristically include sports related activities such as swimming, aerobics, golfing, skiing, and tennis just to name a few.

Fundamentals of Cardiaquatics

The Cardiaquatics Protocol consists of four levels designated by roman numerals. Each level is subdivided into sequences. These sequences are identified with capital letters. Each sequence is further broken down into a series of enumerated activities. These activities are not meant to escalate the patient's heart rate but rather to maintain it within an established range considering the age-adjusted maximal heart rate formula.

In each sequence, the unit of energy or oxygen consumption, the MET, has been taken into consideration, and the estimated amounts have been assigned based on a study of the literature describing similar activities performed on land. The progression of complexity in the applied exercises or activities, particularly in the first three levels, is reflected in the sequence of the three positions used: supine, upright standing, and prone.

Level I consists of three sequences of activities performed in the supine position. Consequently, these will require the use of floatation devices. The approximate METs in this level might range from three to four. The highlight of this level is the third sequence where three Bad Ragaz patterns have been integrated. Manual resistance may be added to selected activities in sequences B and C.

Level II features a program of aquacalisthenics performed in the upright standing position. This level is the lengthiest and for that reason has the widest range of assigned METs, which might begin at 1.5 and progress to 4. Consisting of six sequences, the first three constitute the warm up segment of the Cardiaquatics protocol. The sequences in this second level progress in complexity and exercise intensity. Water depth is an important consideration. A depth of three to four feet is recommended, depending on the patient's height, so the surface of the water is at the xiphoid process.

Monitoring each participant throughout the session continues to be of significant importance in determining whether or not the patient is compliant with the particular level or sequence. Blood pressure and heart rate are recorded at the beginning and end of the session on the Cardiaquatics Flow Sheet (Figure 180). Heart rate is also monitored at regular intervals during the session. If you provide a laminated copy of the Cardiaquatics Flow Sheet and an erasable marker, patients can record their own heart rate during the session, and you can transfer the data to the patient's chart after the session.

Equipment and accessories such as weights, paddles, and boards are used in level II to promote strengthening and enhance cardiopulmonary endurance. Nevertheless, we must also consider the added resistance offered by the hydrostatic pressure of the water. With this in mind, it is advised not to use weights in excess of two pounds in keeping with a more conservative approach.

Level III introduces two prone sequences. In this third level, the primary goal is the attainment of optimal cardiovascular fitness and pulmonary ventilation. This is achieved through integrating vigorous swimming activity into the protocol. The optional use of a mask and snorkel is suggested in order to promote optimal tidal volume.

Finally, level IV consists of the application of the Clinical Wassertanzen Protocol of passive maneuvers. The objective in this level is to improve cardiorespiratory endurance. Consequently, the primary (cardiopulmonary) and secondary (musculoskeletal) breathing mechanisms discussed in Chapter 7 (Clinical Wassertanzen) will also apply in this case. In summary, the primary objectives address improvement in lung capacities and volumes; impact on ventilation, perfusion, and

Cardiaquatics Flow Sheet

Preactivity Heart Rate: _____ Preactivity Blood Pressure: _____					
Date	**Level**	**Sequence**	**Activity**	**HR**	**Comments or Pulmonary Function Reading**

Pre-Wata* Pulmonary Function Readings: ____Insp. Cap. ____% SaO$_2$ ____VC
Post-Wata* Pulmonary Function Readings: ____Insp. Cap. ____% SaO$_2$ ____VC

*Wata = Wassertanzen

Figure 180: Cardiaquatics protocol flow sheet.

diffusion capabilities; improvement in arterial gas exchange; and strengthening of the primary respiratory musculature. The secondary objectives focus on improving muscle fiber contractility, connective tissue elasticity, and the biomechanics of joints.

In order to ascertain the attainment of cardiopulmonary goals, measurement of spirometry, oxygen saturation, and/or vital capacity should be recorded before and after the Wassertanzen session. Concerning the application of Wassertanzen maneuvers, it must be stressed that the patient must be proficient in the three phases of breathing control discussed in Chapter 7, which support the physiologic effects of Wassertanzen on the respiratory system. Once the patient has reached adequate post-expiratory tolerance, he will be ready for more advanced passive submersion maneuvers.

Cardiaquatics Protocol: Level I: Supine Activities

Music optional; easy listening music is suggested.

Take pulse and blood pressure; record on laminated flow sheet with erasable marker.

Sequence I A: Wearing floatation collar or floatation vest plus floatation pelvic belt
(10 repetitions of each) Approx. METS: 3 - 3.5

1. Double knee to chest

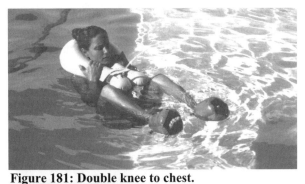

Figure 181: Double knee to chest.

2. Single knee to chest

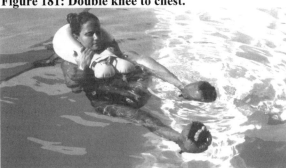

Figure 182: Single knee to chest.

3. Bilateral hip
   abduction

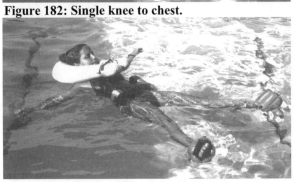

Figure 183: Bilateral hip abduction.

Sequence I A (continued)

4. Bilateral shoulder
   abduction

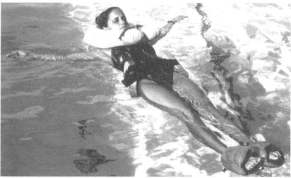

Figure 184: Bilateral shoulder abduction.

5. Reciprocal upper
   extremity overhead
   backwards

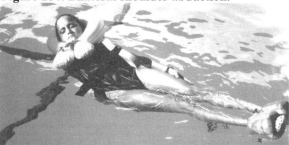

Figure 185: Reciprocal upper extremity overhead backwards.

6. Reciprocal upper
   extremity overhead
   forward

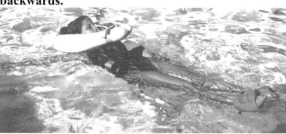

Figure 186: Reciprocal upper extremity overhead forward.

7. Lower extremity
   frog kick with
   simultaneous
   shoulder abduction
   and adduction
   (providing scapular
   support)

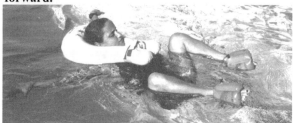

Figure 187: Lower extremity frog kick with simultaneous shoulder abduction and adduction.

Take pulse and record on laminated flow sheet with erasable marker.

Sequence I B: Wearing floatation collar or floatation vest plus floatation pelvic belt
(10 repetitions of each) Approx. METS: 1.5 – 2

1. Unilateral hip and
    shoulder abduction
    and adduction
    (therapist provides
    support at thigh on
    contralateral side;
    then alternate)

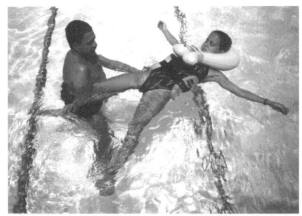

**Figure 188: Unilateral hip and shoulder abduction
and adduction.**

2. Lateral trunk flexion
    (reach for the knee)
    performed
    alternately on each
    side (therapist
    provides hand
    support below head
    of fibula)

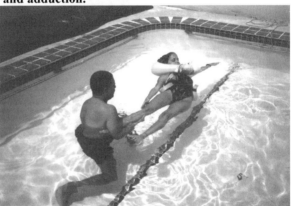

**Figure 189: Lateral trunk flexion performed alter-
nately on each side.**

Take pulse and record on laminated flow sheet with erasable marker.

Sequence I C: Manually Resisted and Isometric Bad Ragaz Patterns (requiring hand placement and facilitation by therapist); wearing a floatation collar or floatation vest plus floatation pelvic belt

        (Repeat 5 times for each side or 10 times bilaterally) Approx. METS: 2 – 3

1. Therapist's command: "Knees straight, toes pointing up, hips up, tighten up your body and don't let me move it to the left hold...hold...hold... relax." (repeat toward the right side). (Isometric Bad Ragaz Pattern)*

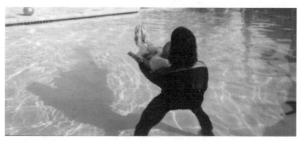

Figure 190: Isometric Bad Ragaz pattern, hand placement is under the scapulae or lateral aspect of thorax.

2. Therapist resists bilateral hip abduction and follows a 360 circle; hand placement is on the lateral aspect of both ankles

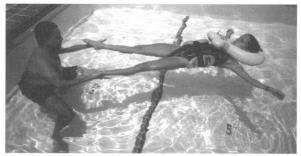

Figure 191: Resisted bilateral simultaneous abduction.

3. Bilateral resisted upper extremity proprioceptive neuromuscular facilitation (PNF) alternating sides; hand placement should switch from dorsal to palmar aspect of hands (Bilateral Upper Extremity Bad Ragaz Pattern, see Figure 96 to Figure 98)*

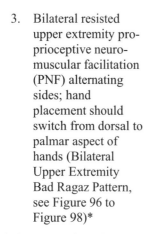

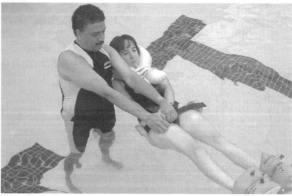

Figure 192: Beginning of the bilateral upper extremity Bad Ragaz pattern.

*The Isometric and Bilateral Upper Extremity Bad Ragaz Patterns are discussed and illustrated in Chapter 4.

Take pulse and record on laminated flow sheet with erasable marker.

Cardiaquatics Protocol: Level II: Aquacalisthenics Standing

Use music as incentive; pop or rock music is highly suggested.

Sequence II A:

(5 repetitions of each. Approx. METS: 1.5 – 2)

1. Four steps forward; four steps sideways to the right; four steps backward; four steps to the left, or the four-corner pivot gait

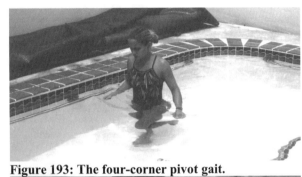

Figure 193: The four-corner pivot gait.

2. Unilateral hip circumduction (leg circles)

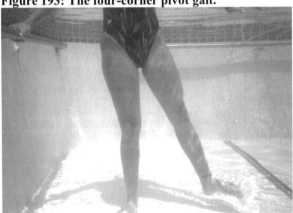

Figure 194: Unilateral hip circumduction in the standing position.

3. Unilateral hip abduction and adduction

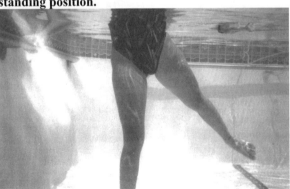

Figure 195: Unilateral hip abduction and adduction.

Sequence II A (continued):

4. Unilateral Lower
   Extremity "Figure 8"

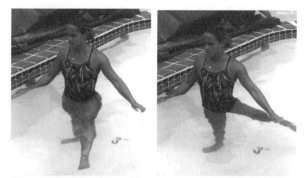

Figure 196: Unilateral lower extremity "figure 8."

5. The Can-Can:
   Unilateral Hip and
   Knee Flexion, then,
   hyper-extension of
   hip with extension of
   knee

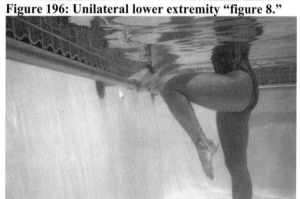

Figure 197: The Can-Can: unilateral hip and knee flexion...

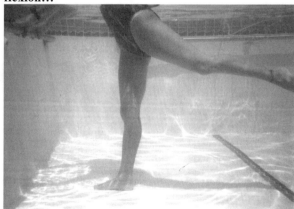

Figure 198: ...and hyperextension of hip with extension of knee.

Take pulse and record on laminated flow sheet with erasable marker.

Sequence II B: Using board

(10 repetitions of each. Approx. METS: 2 - 2.5)

1. Hold board horizontally, push down, straightening out elbows, and release

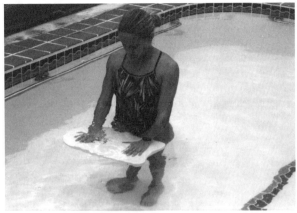

Figure 199: Pushing down on board from standing position.

2. Hold board vertically and rotate trunk to the right; then, return to the original position and release

3. Hold board vertically and rotate trunk to the left; then, return to the original position and release

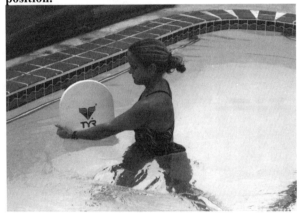

Figure 200: Rotating trunk with board.

Take pulse and record on laminated flow sheet with erasable marker.

Sequence II C: Holding paddles vertically in each hand*, elbows slightly bent; right or left foot forward (then switch)

(10 repetitions of each. Approx. METS: 2 – 3)

1. Push down and horizontally abduct shoulder

2. Push down and horizontally adduct shoulder

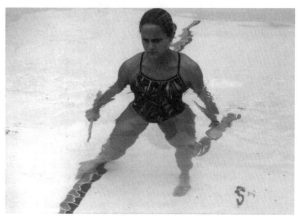

Figure 201: Horizontally abducting and adducting shoulders using paddles.

3. Push down and hyperextend shoulder; then, flex shoulder to 90°

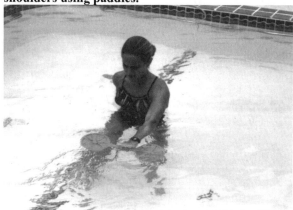

Figure 202: Hyperextending and flexing shoulder using paddles.

*Degree of resistance in paddles can be adjusted for more or less resistance.

Take pulse and record on laminated flow sheet with erasable marker.

Sequence II D: Holding aqua-dumbbells bilaterally, bend elbows and knees slightly
(Complete 5 - 10 laps of each. Approx. METS: 3 - 3.5)

1. Forward walk
    swinging arms
    alternately with
    elbows extended
    (water level at
    xiphoid process)

2. Forward walk
    swinging arms
    alternately with
    reciprocal flexion and
    extension (water level
    at midsternum)

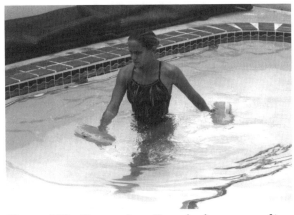

Figure 203: Forward walk swinging arms alternately with elbows extended, using aqua-dumbbells.

3. Forward walk with
    bilateral shoulder
    abduction and
    adduction

Take pulse and record on laminated flow sheet with erasable marker.

Sequence II E:
(10 - 20 repetitions of each, or 5 - 10 minutes in activity #3. Approx. METS: 2.5 - 3.5)

1. Reciprocal Hip-
    Reach-and-Jump

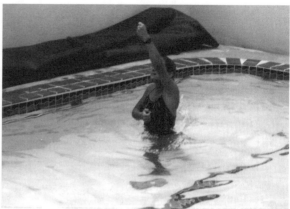

Figure 204: Reciprocal hip-reach-and-jump

2. Hoola hoop circle
    walking

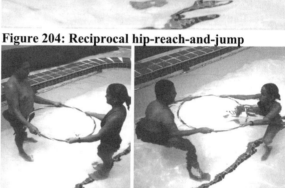

Figure 205: The hoola hoop circle walk activity.

3. Water volleyball
    (infinity ball); or,
    scuba ball as an
    alternative

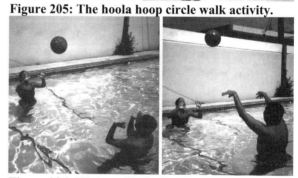

Figure 206: Water volleyball.

Take pulse and record on laminated flow sheet with erasable marker.

Sequence II F: Using the AquaJogger or tether apparatus in 6 to 8 feet of water depth, (20 - 50 repetitions of each. Approx. METS: 3 – 4)

1. Bicycle or jog for 2 - 5 minutes without ankle weights

2. Bicycle or jog for 2 - 5 minutes using 2 lbs ankle weights

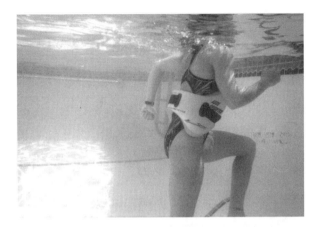

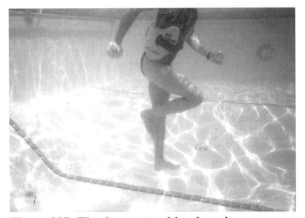

Figure 207: The deep-water bicycle or jog.

Take pulse and record on laminated flow sheet with erasable marker.

Cardiaquatics Protocol: Level III: Prone Activities
No music

Sequence III A: Wearing mask and snorkel plus floatation gear as needed
(Complete 3 round trip laps. Approx. METS: 2 - 2.5)

1. Modified breaststroke
    (maintain head in
    neutral)

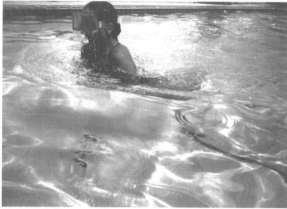

Figure 208: Modified breaststroke using mask and snorkel.

2. Upper body
    swimming (moving
    arms reciprocally or
    bilaterally while
    kicking legs);
    coordinate deep
    breathing with
    activity

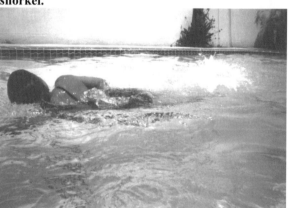

Figure 209: Upper body swimming with reciprocal arm movement and leg kicks.

Take pulse and record on laminated flow sheet with erasable marker.

Sequence III B: Wearing floatation gear as needed

(Approx. METS; 4 – 5)

1. Swim one lap across one way; then rest for 1 minute and swim another lap returning to the point of origin

2. Swim one round trip of laps; rest for 1 minute and swim another round trip

3. Swim five round trips laps; rest for 5 minutes and repeat activity. Alternative activity: Interval training with tether apparatus

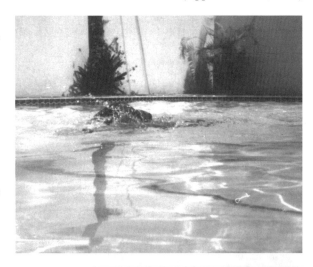

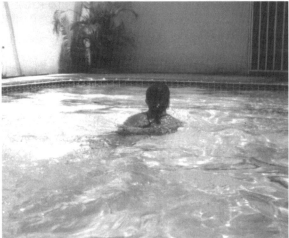

Figure 210: Swimming laps.

Take pulse and record on laminated flow sheet with erasable marker.

Cardiaquatics Protocol: Level IV: Clinical Wassertanzen
Music should be used as an incentive to enhance relaxation

Measure Inspiratory Capacity with an inspirometer, or O_2 Saturation with an oximeter (see Figure 211), or Forced Vital Capacity

Objectives:
- improve vital capacity, tidal volume, expiratory reserve volume, and inspiratory capacity
- improve ventilation, perfusion, and diffusion capabilities of the lungs
- improve the mobility of the spine and weight-bearing joints
- improve the function of the diaphragm and intercostal muscles
- induce a state of relaxation
- reduce muscle tension

Considerations:
Practitioner must have undergone training and certification on the Clinical Wassertanzen Protocol. The practitioner must further be trained and experience in the theory and skill. It is fundamentally important for the patient to be trained in and proficient in practicing the three phases of breathing control featured in the Clinical Wassertanzen Protocol. These are
1. Breathing control in the upright position
2. Breathing control in the supine position
3. Breathing control in submersions

All principles of breathing should be explained to the patient. The therapist should be selective to be sure that he integrates applied passive maneuvers and integrated manual techniques that will best benefit the patient. It is not necessary to apply the entire protocol. It is best to be selective until the patient is proficient enough in the third phase of breathing control and can tolerate the entire progression.

Protocol:
Phase I
1. Tidal volume and vital capacity retraining
2. Post expiratory endurance (3 stages)
3. Water breath dance

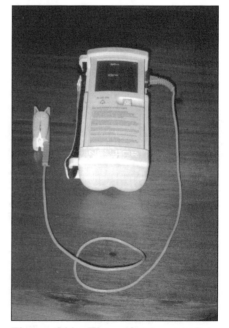

Figure 211: The oximeter used to measure oxygen saturation levels.

Phase II
1. Applied lateral sacral glides
2. Applied soft tissue and myofascial releases
3. Trigger point releases
4. Cervical spine distraction
5. Cradled rocking

Phase III
1. Passive full body flexion
2. Passive maneuver of the pelvic belt musculature with proximal hold
3. Passive maneuver of the pelvic belt musculature with distal hold
4. Passive pelvic and spine rotations
5. Prone spine snaking maneuver
6. Passive thoracolumbar flexion-extension
7. Scapulohumeral distraction
8. Scapulothoracic mobilization
9. Cervico-thoraco-lumbar spine rotations
10. Lumbosacral and pelvic stabilization with integrated tibiofemoral joint approximation and actebulofemoral anteroposterior glides
11. Passive full body flexion
12. Watsu® Sequence: Bilateral repetitive

Measure Inspiratory Capacity with an inspirometer, or O_2 Saturation with an oximeter, or Forced Vital Capacity

Conclusion

The Cardiaquatics protocol consists of a four-level, multi-sequence program of aquatic activities and exercises designed for the patient known to have cardiac problems (with prior cardiac rehabilitation on land), for the patient with documented risk factors, or for patients with general deconditioning. The integrated activities within the levels and sequences allow the clinician to select those that are most appropriate for his patients considering the patient's history, state of physical health, and associated medical problems.

Cardiaquatics focuses on improving cardiovascular fitness and muscular strength in addition to improving pulmonary ventilation, perfusion, and diffusion.

Section III

Clinical Applications

CHAPTER 9

CARDIOPULMONARY APPLICATIONS

Emphysema

The main problem experienced by a patient with emphysema is loss of the elastic recoil properties of the lungs due to bronchiolar distention, particularly in patients diagnosed with panlobular emphysema. Destruction of the respiratory bronchiole accompanied by edema and inflammation is a clinical finding in patients with centrilobular emphysema. Distention of the pulmonary tissue leads to dyspnea and reflects in the type of hypoxemia that is characteristic of the patient with emphysema.

These patients appear very thin and present with an increased A-P (antero-posterior) diameter of the chest. Bi-basilar excursions are extremely compromised due to recruitment of and dependency on the accessory muscles of respiration. However, most patients with emphysema are "dry." This implies that they do not exhibit a produc-

tive cough. Lung auscultation generally indicates diminished or absents breath sounds throughout the bilateral lung fields. This depends on the extent or severity of the disease, e.g., end-stage emphysema.

The hydrostatic pressure of the water exerts resistance against the external thoracic wall. This property serves as a means for strengthening and re-educating the intercostal musculature and diaphragm. The objective is to strengthen these primary respiratory muscles so that the patient has less need to utilize the accessory muscles, namely, the sternocleidomastoid and scalenes.

Activities in the upright position are most important before one considers integrating other interventions in the supine position. The therapist should begin with basic aquatic activities such as relaxation techniques that incorporate lateral costal and basal exercises and diaphragmatic breathing. Segmental breathing exercises can be gradually

173

included in the protocol of aquatic activities. If the patient is oxygen-dependent, he must perform the activities while connected to the oxygen source. Provisions should be made for an extralong connecting tube so that gait and other aquatic activities are not interrupted because of insufficiently long tubing. The patient should be able to move freely throughout the pool without fear of disconnecting the oxygen source. Oximetry should be monitored prior to and after the aquatic therapy session and at regular intervals during the session to make sure that the patient is not desaturating significantly.

The preaquatic evaluation of the patient with emphysema places emphasis on thoracic auscultation, thoracic symmetry, and assessment of diaphragmatic and costolateral breathing. Review of the patient's chest x-ray and arterial blood gases provides the therapist with further insight into the patient's status. The chest x-ray might reveal predisposition to the development of pulmonary bullae. Pulmonary bullae are bubbled, balloon-like formations on the surface or periphery of the lung parenchyma as a result of alveolar distention. When present, these pulmonary bullae might burst, placing the patient in imminent danger of developing a pneumothorax. If the patient exhibits a productive cough, it is advised to wait until lung fields are cleared of secretions before beginning aquatic therapy.

The aquatic therapy plan of care for the patient with emphysema must focus on the integration of energy conservation techniques. Metered ambulation in the pool is strongly recommended with assistance and close monitoring. Adapted Halliwick armhold techniques will provide the desired level of assistance during this activity. Stair climbing is not recommended be-

cause it places an increased demand on the patient's cardiovascular and pulmonary systems, and will result in early fatigue with dyspnea on exertion. Keeping in mind that patients with emphysema have a low endurance and can maintain minimally adequate blood gases, the therapist must carefully design and select activities to avoid risking further respiratory complications. Transfer of the patient in and out of the pool should be carried out via a hydraulic lift device. A bench should be provided for the patient to sit on once he is transferred into the pool.

Once the patient has adjusted to the environment and mastered activities in the upright sitting position, other interventions in the supine position requiring application of floatation equipment may be integrated. These can include segmental breathing exercises and selected Bad Ragaz patterns such as the bilateral upper extremity, unilateral upper extremity, and passive trunk elongation with thoracic hold. The latter focuses on reeducation of the intercostal musculature utilizing the stretch reflex as the facilitation technique to elicit bucket-handle thoracic mobility. Selected Watsu® basic and transitional flow movement sequences would be effective in promoting relaxation and improving breathing dynamics.

Emphysema Case Study

The following emphysema case utilizes the DASI pre-aquatic assessment form to present clinical findings, establish goals, and select the interventions that would best meet the established goals. A discussion of the case is provided to justify the selection of activities, techniques, and interventions and to suggest other potentially effective strategies in the clinical management of a patient with emphysema.

DASI
Diagnostic Aquatics Systems Integration — Pre-Aquatic Therapy Assessment

Patient Name: _____*Joe*_____   Date: _____

Dx: ___*Emphysema*_____   Age: ___*54*_____

History/Problems/Complaints: *Pt presents with a 4-year hx of panlobular emphysema. O_2 dependent @ 3L via nasal cannulas. Recent ABG's: pO_2=88 pCO_2=55 pH=7.21 HCO_3=20 SaO_2=90%. Evidence of dyspnea and tachypnea. Moderate cyanosis noted. CXR shows evidence of distended lungs with bilaterally flattened diaphragm.*
Clinical Impression: *Severe functional decline; severe deconditioning; significantly decreased endurance*

Musculoskeletal Assessment

Musculoskeletal Assessment		Manual Muscle Test		Range of Motion	
		Right	Left	Right	Left
Shoulder	Flexors	3+/5	3+/5	160°	145°
	Extensors	3+/5	3+/5	WFL	WFL
	Abductors	3+/5	3+/5	150°	140°
	Adductors	3+/5	3+/5	WFL	WFL
	External Rotators	3+/5	3+/5	30°	25°
	Internal Rotators	3+/5	3+/5	20°	20°
Elbow	Flexors	4/5	4/5	WFL	WFL
	Extensors	4-/5	4-/5	WFL	WFL
Forearm	Pronators	4/5	4/5	WFL	WFL
	Supinators	4/5	4/5	WFL	WFL
Wrist	Flexors	4-/5	4-/5	WFL	WFL
	Extensors	4-/5	4-/5	WFL	WFL
Finger	Flexors/Hand Grip	3/5	3/5	WFL	WFL
Hip	Flexors	3/5	3/5	WFL	WFL
	Extensors	3/5	3/5	10°	10°
	Abductors	3/5	3/5	WFL	WFL
	Adductors	3/5	3/5	WFL	WFL
	External Rotators	3/5	3/5	WFL	WFL
	Internal Rotators	3/5	3/5	WFL	WFL

Musculoskeletal Assessment		Manual Muscle Test		Range of Motion	
		Right	Left	Right	Left
Knee	Flexors	3/5	3/5	WFL	WFL
	Extensors	3+/5	3+/5	WFL	WFL
Ankle	Dorsiflexors	4-/5	4-/5	WFL	WFL
	Plantar Flexors	4/5	4/5	WFL	WFL
Foot	Invertors	4-	4-/5	WFL	WFL
	Evertors	4-/:	4-/5	WFL	WFL

Musculoskeletal Assessment	ROM	MMT
Cervical Flexion	WFL	4+/5
Cervical Extension	10°	4-/5
Cervical Lateral Flexion (right)	5°	4/5
Cervical Lateral Flexion (left)	5°	4/5
Cervical Rotation (right)	5°	4/5
Cervical Rotation (left)	5°	4/5
Lumbar Flexion	WFL	4/5
Lumbar Extension	WFL	4/5
Lumbar Lateral Flexion (right)	WFL	4/5
Lumbar Lateral Flexion (left)	WFL	4/5

Evidence of Edema? ☐ Yes   ■ No

Girth Anatomical Landmark: _____ ■ Not Applicable

Right: _____ inch(es)   Left: _____ inch(es)

Leg-Length Discrepancy?   ☐ Yes   ■ No
Approximate Discrepancy: _____ inch(es)

Musculoskeletal Assessment (continued)

Posture

		Explain
Posture	☐ Normal Alignment ■ Postural Deviations	*Pigeon chest deformity*

Spasmodic Activity

		Grade			
	☐ No evidence of muscle spasms ☐ Not applicable	**1**	**2**	**3**	**4**
Spasmodic Activity	**Muscles**				
	rt SCM				■
	lt SCM				■

Cardiopulmonary Assessment

Cardiopulmonary Assessment

Lungs	☐ Clear to Auscultation ■ Abnormal Breath Sounds *Diminished bibasilar breath sounds* ☐ Adventitious Breath Sounds ☐ Resonant Chest to Mediate Percussion ■ Other: *Hyperresonance* ■ Bibasilar Thoracic Asymmetry *Decreased bibasilar, increased biapical* RR: *32/min* ☐ Normal ■ Dyspnea ☐ Other:
Cardiac	☐ Normal S1 Other: ■ Normal S2 ■ Split S1 ☐ Split S2 ☐ S3 ☐ S4 ☐ Murmur ☐ Ejection Click HR: _____ BP: _____

Neurological Assessment

Neurologic Assessment	
Superficial Sensation	■ Intact Explain ☐ Impaired
Coordination	■ Intact Explain ☐ Impaired ☐ Intention Tremors
Proprioception	■ Intact Explain ☐ Impaired
Deep Tendon Reflexes	■ Intact Explain ☐ Diminished _____ ☐ Hyperactive _____
Balance	Static ■ Intact ☐ Impaired Dynamic ☐ Intact ■ Impaired

	No Pain Intolerable Pain
Pain	■ 1 2 3 4 5 6 7 8 9 10
Tone	■ Normal ☐ Hypertonia / Spasticity ☐ Hypotonia / Flaccidity ☐ Cogwheel Rigidity ☐ Contractures

	Check the Appropriate Box			
		Pos	**Neg**	**N/A**
Other Neurologic Test Results	SLR Test	☐	☐	■
	Neural Tension	☐	☐	■
	Ulnar Radial Median			
	Fabere Sign	☐	☐	■
	Compression Test	☐	☐	■
	Distraction Stretch	☐	☐	■
	Vertebral Artery Test	☐	☐	■
	Alar Ligament Test	☐	☐	■
	Vertebral Glide Test	☐	☐	■
	Babinski Sign	☐	☐	■
	Romberg's Test	☐	☐	■
	Other	☐	☐	■

Functional Assessment

	Mobility
Gait Analysis	■ Ambulatory ❏ Non-Ambulatory Explain: ■ Assistive Device: *Rolling Walker* Weight Bearing: ■ FWB ❏ PWB ❏ NWB ❏ No significant gait deviations noted. ❏ Gait Deviations: ■ Abnormal Gait *Bilateral shuffle w/ decreased ankle dorsiflexion*
Bed Mobility	■ Independent ❏ Requires assistance ❏ max ❏ mod ❏ min
Transfers	■ Independent ❏ Requires assistance ❏ max ❏ mod ❏ min
Body Mechanics	■ Not tested ❏ Uses proper body mechanics when lifting, carrying, sitting, and lying down ❏ Does not use proper body mechanics when lifting, carrying, and lying down ❏ Needs further instruction and practice

Goals

■ Improve endurance
■ Improve balance
❏ Improve spinal mobility
❏ Promote relaxation
■ Improve breathing patterns
Diaphragmatic and costolateral
❏ Decrease pain
_____

❏ Increase muscle strength
_____

❏ Increase joint range and flexibility
_____

■ Improve gait pattern
❏ Improve coordination and proprioception
❏ Reduce muscle fatigue
❏ Decrease edema and inflammation
_____

❏ Improve postural alignment
❏ Improve circulation
❏ Improve motor control
❏ Inhibit spasticity/hypertonicity
_____

■ Resolution of muscle spasms:
bilateral SCM
_____

Plan of Care

Frequency: __3__ times per week for __4__ weeks

Bad Ragaz	■ Passive Relaxation ❏ Passive Pelvic Tilts ❏ Pre-Gait ❏ Isotonic #1 ❏ Isotonic #2 ❏ Isometric ❏ Pre-Weight-Bearing ❏ Tone Inhibition ❏ Passive Trunk Elongation/Knee Hold ❏ Passive Trunk Elongation/Pelvic Hold ■ Passive Trunk Elongation/Thoracic Hold ■ Unilateral Upper Extremity ■ Bilateral Upper Extremity ❏ Prone Unilateral Upper Extremity ❏ Unilateral Lower Extremity ❏ Bilateral Lower Extremity ❏ Bilateral Symmetrical Lower Extremity #1 ❏ Bilateral Symmetrical Lower Extremity #2 ❏ Bilateral Reciprocal Lower Extremity ❏ Other:
Halliwick	❏ Phase I Adjustment ❏ Phase II Rotational Activities ❏ Turbulent Gliding ❏ Balance Training/Kangaroo Jumps ❏ Balance Training/Weight Shifting ■ Other: *Halliwick breathing activities w/ flip balls*

Cardiaquatics	❏ Level I Sequences: ____ Activities: ____
	❏ Level II Sequences: ____ Activities: ____
	❏ Level III Sequences: ____ Activities: ____
	❏ Level IV
	      ❏ Phase 1 ❏ Phase 2 ❏ Phase 3 ❏ All
	      ❏ Selected Sequences:

Other	❏ Applied Myofascial Release ❏ Deep Friction Massage ❏ Applied Joint Mobilization/Distraction ❏ Applied Spinal Mobilization/Distraction ❏ Applied Joint Approximation ❏ Applied Feldenkrais ❏ Applied Lymphatic Drainage ■ Watsu/Basic Flow ■ Watsu/Transitional Flow ■ Clinical Wassertanzen I ❏ Clinical Wassertanzen II ❏ Clinical Wassertanzen III ❏ Applied Aquatic Craniosacral Therapy ❏ Trigger Point Therapy ❏ Ai Chi: _____ ❏ Spinal/Trunk Stabilization Protocol: _____ ❏ Thoracic Outlet Syndrome Protocol: _____ ❏ Other:

Functional / Goal Specific Aquatic Therapy Activities and Exercises

■ Gait Training (Forward/Backward) Laps: *1-3*
❏ Stair Climbing x ____
❏ Bicycling Reps: ____
❏ Prone Activities Min ____
❏ Aquajogging Laps: ____
❏ Heel Cord Stretch
❏ Iliopsoas Stretch
❏ Piriformis Stretch
❏ TFL Stretch
❏ IT Band Stretch
❏ Hip Add Stretch
❏ Stork Stand
❏ Front to Back Weight Shifting
❏ Side to Side Weight Shifting
❏ Heel Raises Reps: ____
❏ Four-Corner Pivot Reps: ____

❏ Side-Stepping Laps: ____
❏ Cross Over Stepping Laps: ____
❏ Deep-Water Stride Jump Reps: ____
■ Deep-Water Jogging (fwd/retro): 5 min.
❏ Deep-Water Groin Stretch
❏ Knee to Chest Reps: ____
❏ Closed Kinematic Chain Exercises
❏ Deep-Water Double Knee Lifts Reps: ____
❏ Wall Slide Reps: ____
❏ Pelvic Tilts Reps: ____
❏ Supine Kicks Reps: ____
❏ Deep-Water Spinal Traction in Vertical Suspension
(____ lbs. x ____ min.)
❏ Resistive Exercises:

■ Other: *Metered ambulation in shallow water with oximetry*

Aquatic Work Conditioning

❏ Resistive Forward/Retro Gait x ____ laps
❏ Deep-Water Jogging (fwd/retro) x ____ min.
❏ Tethered Jogging # ____ x ____ min.
❏ Swimming: ____ laps/min

❏ Other:

Equipment Used

■ Bodyfit® Collar
❏ Floatation Vest
❏ Tire Tube
■ Floatation Pelvic Belt
❏ Fins
❏ Snorkel Mask
❏ Snorkel Tube
❏ Ankle Floats
❏ Aqua-Dumbbells

❏ AquaJogger
❏ Graduated-Resistance Paddles
❏ Hydrotone Boots
❏ Hoola Hoop
❏ Resistance Cord
❏ Thera-Band®
❏ Aquakinetic Machines
❏ Boards
❏ Floatation Noodle

❏ Hydrotone Dumbbells
❏ Weights: ____
■ Bad Ragaz Floatation Rings
❏ Swim Bar
❏ Recumbent Bicycle
❏ Underwater Treadmill
■ Halliwick Blow Balls
❏ Other:_____

Adjunct Therapy

■ Not Applicable

❏ Whirlpool: ____ min. (spa)
❏ Patient Education
❏ Posture and Body Mechanics
❏ Home Exercise Program

❏ Other:_____

Land Based Therapy Treatments

■ Not Applicable

Frequency: ____ times per week
for ____ weeks
❏ US: _____
❏ ES: _____
❏ HP's: _____
❏ Massage: _____

❏ Therapeutic Exercises (specify):
❏ Paraffin Bath:
❏ Cryotherapy:
❏ Joint Mobilization:
❏ Piriformis Release

Comments:
Monitor O₂ saturation level at regular intervals during and between each intervention or activity
Maintain O₂ therapy @ 3L via nasal cannulas during shallow-water dynamic activities and all aquatic therapy interventions using extended connecting tube to allow mobility in the water

_____   _____
Signature & Credentials of Therapist   Date

Discussion

Based on the documented clinical findings, the interventions selected in the plan of care for this case are aimed at improving chest excursions and strengthening the intercostal musculature through applied stretch reflex facilitation. Additionally, selected activities include those focused on energy conservation and prevention of excessive fatigue. Considering the documented values on the arterial blood gases, oximetry monitoring is highly recommended. Clinical manifestations must also be considered. If the patient is severely dyspneic, he might not tolerate even the mildest of activities. Sometimes it is best to begin with tolerance and adjustment using hydrostatic pressure as the conduit. The patient should simply sit on a chair in shallow water for a determined period of time while monitored by the aquatic therapist. Besides the observations of clinical signs that might suggest inability to tolerate this activity, oximetry should be another monitoring technique integrated into the activity. Generalized deconditioning associated with the respiratory problems is noticeable throughout the manual muscle test. Documented limitations of joint range might be associated with the patient's difficulty in moving an extremity against gravity. In the cervical region, there is evidence of increased use of the sternocleidomastoid muscle as the primary accessory muscle. This evidence is justified in increased myofibril activity and presence of spasmodic activity along with limited range of the antagonists.

Asthma

The patient with asthma experiences a widespread narrowing of the airway secondary to bronchospasm. From an anatomical basis, the mucosa of the airway is inflamed with hyperactive goblet cells, which produce increased amounts of exudate. The degree of bronchospastic disease is reflected by the presence of wheezes during auscultation. The primary clinical problem for a patient with asthma is a poor vital capacity due to airway shunting as a result of bronchospasms during the expiratory phase. This leads to weakness of the primary respiratory musculature and reliance on the use of the accessory muscles. Subsequently, hypoxemia and hypercarbia will also characterize these patients.

Asthma Case Study

The following asthma case utilizes the DASI pre-aquatic assessment form to present clinical findings, establish goals, and select the interventions that would best meet the established goals. A discussion of the case is provided to justify the selection of activities, techniques, and interventions and to suggest other potentially effective strategies in the clinical management of the patient with asthma. Any type of aquatic therapy intervention is contraindicated in acute status asthmaticus.

DASI
Diagnostic Aquatics Systems Integration — Pre-Aquatic Therapy Assessment

Patient Name: _____*Mary*_____ Date: _____

Dx: __*Asthma*_____ Age: ___*40*_____

History/Problems/Complaints: *ABG's: pO_2=90 pCO_2=61 pH=7.18 HCO_3=21 SaO_2=92%. Evidence of dyspnea and tachypnea. CXR shows alveolar infiltrates.*
Clinical Impression: *Functional decline with deconditioning; decreased endurance*

Musculoskeletal Assessment

Musculoskeletal Assessment		Manual Muscle Test		Range of Motion	
		Right	Left	Right	Left
Shoulder	Flexors	4+/5	4+/5	WFL	WFL
	Extensors	4+/5	4+/5	WFL	WFL
	Abductors	4+/5	4+/5	WFL	WFL
	Adductors	4+/5	4+/5	WFL	WFL
	External Rotators	4+/5	4+/5	WFL	WFL
	Internal Rotators	4+/5	4+/5	WFL	WFL
Elbow	Flexors	4/5	4/5	WFL	WFL
	Extensors	4/5	4/5	WFL	WFL
Forearm	Pronators	4/5	4/5	WFL	WFL
	Supinators	4/5	4/5	WFL	WFL
Wrist	Flexors	4/5	4/5	WFL	WFL
	Extensors	4/5	4/5	WFL	WFL
Finger	Flexors/Hand Grip	3+/5	3+/5	WFL	WFL
Hip	Flexors	4-/5	4-/5	WFL	WFL
	Extensors	3+/5	3+/5	WFL	WFL
	Abductors	3+/5	3+/5	WFL	WFL
	Adductors	3+/5	3+/5	WFL	WFL
	External Rotators	4/5	4/5	WFL	WFL
	Internal Rotators	4/5	4/5	WFL	WFL

Musculoskeletal Assessment		Manual Muscle Test		Range of Motion	
		Right	Left	Right	Left
Knee	Flexors	4/5	4/5	WFL	WFL
	Extensors	4+/5	4+/5	WFL	WFL
Ankle	Dorsiflexors	4/5	4/5	WFL	WFL
	Plantar Flexors	4/5	4/5	WFL	WFL
Foot	Invertors	4/5	4/5	WFL	WFL
	Evertors	4/5	4/5	WFL	WFL

Musculoskeletal Assessment		ROM	MMT
Spine	Cervical Flexion	WFL	4+/5
	Cervical Extension	10°	4/5
	Cervical Lateral Flexion (right)	10°	4/5
	Cervical Lateral Flexion (left)	10°	4/5
	Cervical Rotation (right)	10°	4/5
	Cervical Rotation (left)	10°	4/5
	Lumbar Flexion	WFL	4/5
	Lumbar Extension	WFL	4/5
	Lumbar Lateral Flexion (right)	WFL	4/5
	Lumbar Lateral Flexion (left)	WFL	4/5

Evidence of Edema? ☐ Yes ■ No

Girth Anatomical Landmark: _____ ■ Not Applicable			
Right:	_____inch(es)	Left:	_____ inch(es)

Leg-Length Discrepancy? ☐ Yes ■ No
Approximate Discrepancy: _____ inch(es)

Musculoskeletal Assessment (continued)

Posture

Posture		
❏ Normal Alignment ■ Postural Deviations	**Explain** *Barrel chest deformity*	

Spasmodic Activity

❏ No evidence of muscle spasms ❏ Not applicable	**Grade**			
	1	**2**	**3**	**4**

	Muscles	1	2	3	4
Spasmodic Activity	rt SCM				■
	lt SCM				■
	Scalenes		■		

Cardiopulmonary Assessment

Cardiopulmonary Assessment

Lungs

❏ Clear to Auscultation
■ Abnormal Breath Sounds
Respiratory wheezes BLL and RML
❏ Adventitious Breath Sounds

❏ Resonant Chest to Mediate Percussion
■ Other: *Hypersonant*
■ Bibasilar Thoracic Asymmetry
Decreased bibasilar; increased biapical

RR: *28/min*   ❏ Normal ❏ Dyspnea ❏ Other:

Cardiac

❏ Normal S1 ■ Normal S2 ■ Split S1 ❏ Split S2 ❏ S3 ❏ S4 ❏ Murmur ❏ Ejection Click HR: _____ BP: _____	Other:

Neurological Assessment

Neurologic Assessment

Superficial Sensation	■ Intact ❏ Impaired	**Explain**
Coordination	■ Intact ❏ Impaired ❏ Intention Tremors	**Explain**
Proprioception	■ Intact ❏ Impaired	**Explain**
Deep Tendon Reflexes	■ Intact ❏ Diminished _____ ❏ Hyperactive _____	**Explain**
Balance	Static ■ Intact ❏ Impaired Dynamic ■ Intact ❏ Impaired	

Pain

No Pain   Intolerable Pain
■ 1 2 3 4 5 6 7 8 9 10

Tone

■ Normal
❏ Hypertonia / Spasticity
❏ Hypotonia / Flaccidity
❏ Cogwheel Rigidity
❏ Contractures

Other Neurologic Test Results

	Check the Appropriate Box		
	Pos	Neg	N/A
SLR Test	❏	❏	■
Neural Tension	❏	❏	■
	Ulnar	Radial	Median
Fabere Sign	❏	❏	■
Compression Test	❏	❏	■
Distraction Stretch	❏	❏	■
Vertebral Artery Test	❏	❏	■
Alar Ligament Test	❏	❏	■
Vertebral Glide Test	❏	❏	■
Babinski Sign	❏	❏	■
Romberg's Test	❏	❏	■
Other	❏	❏	■

Functional Assessment

Mobility		
Gait Analysis	■ Ambulatory ☐Non-Ambulatory Explain: ☐ Assistive Device: Weight Bearing: ■ FWB ☐ PWB ☐ NWB ☐ No significant gait deviations noted. ☐ Gait Deviations: ☐ Abnormal Gait	
Bed Mobility	■ Independent ☐ Requires assistance ☐ max ☐ mod ☐ min	
Transfers	■ Independent ☐ Requires assistance ☐ max ☐ mod ☐ min	
Body Mechanics	■ Not tested ☐ Uses proper body mechanics when lifting, carrying, sitting, and lying down ☐ Does not use proper body mechanics when lifting, carrying, and lying down ☐ Needs further instruction and practice	

Goals

■ Improve endurance
☐ Improve balance
☐ Improve spinal mobility
☐ Promote relaxation
■ Improve breathing patterns
Diaphragmatic and costolateral
☐ Decrease pain
_____

☐ Increase muscle strength
_____

☐ Increase joint range and flexibility
_____

☐ Improve gait pattern
☐ Improve coordination and proprioception
☐ Reduce muscle fatigue
☐ Decrease edema and inflammation
_____

☐ Improve postural alignment
☐ Improve circulation
☐ Improve motor control
☐ Inhibit spasticity/hypertonicity
_____

■ Resolution of muscle spasms:
SCM and scalenes
_____

Plan of Care

Frequency: _3__ times per week for _4___ weeks

Bad Ragaz	■ Passive Relaxation ☐ Passive Pelvic Tilts ☐ Pre-Gait ☐ Isotonic #1 ☐ Isotonic #2 ☐ Isometric ☐ Pre-Weight-Bearing ☐ Tone Inhibition ☐ Passive Trunk Elongation/Knee Hold ☐ Passive Trunk Elongation/Pelvic Hold ■ Passive Trunk Elongation/Thoracic Hold ■ Unilateral Upper Extremity ■ Bilateral Upper Extremity ☐ Prone Unilateral Upper Extremity ☐ Unilateral Lower Extremity ☐ Bilateral Lower Extremity ☐ Bilateral Symmetrical Lower Extremity #1 ☐ Bilateral Symmetrical Lower Extremity #2 ☐ Bilateral Reciprocal Lower Extremity ■ Other: *Pelvic trunk elongation with elbow hold*
Halliwick	☐ Phase I Adjustment ☐ Phase II Rotational Activities ☐ Turbulent Gliding ☐ Balance Training/Kangaroo Jumps ☐ Balance Training/Weight Shifting ■ Other: *Halliwick breathing activities with flip balls*
Cardiaquatics	☐ Level I Sequences: _____ Activities: ____ ☐ Level II Sequences: ____ Activities: ____ ☐ Level III Sequences: _____ Activities: ____ ☐ Level IV ☐ Phase 1 ☐ Phase 2 ☐ Phase 3 ☐ All ☐ Selected Sequences:
Other	☐ Applied Myofascial Release ☐ Deep Friction Massage ☐ Applied Joint Mobilization/Distraction ☐ Applied Spinal Mobilization/Distraction ☐ Applied Joint Approximation ☐ Applied Feldenkrais ☐ Applied Lymphatic Drainage ■ Watsu/Basic Flow ■ Watsu/Transitional Flow ■ Clinical Wassertanzen I ■ Clinical Wassertanzen II ☐ Clinical Wassertanzen III ☐ Applied Aquatic Craniosacral Therapy ☐ Trigger Point Therapy ■ Ai Chi: *Upper extremity exercises* ☐ Spinal/Trunk Stabilization Protocol: _____ ☐ Thoracic Outlet Syndrome Protocol: _____ ☐ Other: _____

Functional / Goal Specific Aquatic Therapy Activities and Exercises

■ Gait Training (Forward/Backward) Laps: *1-3*
❏ Stair Climbing x ____
❏ Bicycling Reps: ____
■ Prone Activities Min *3*
❏ Aquajogging Laps: ____
❏ Heal Cord Stretch
❏ Iliopsoas Stretch
❏ Piriformis Stretch
❏ TFL Stretch
❏ IT Band Stretch
❏ Hip Add Stretch
❏ Stork Stand
❏ Front to Back Weight Shifting
❏ Side to Side Weight Shifting
❏ Heel Raises Reps: ____
❏ Four-Corner Pivot Reps: ____

❏ Side-Stepping Laps: ____
❏ Cross Over Stepping Laps: ____
❏ Deep-Water Stride Jump Reps: ____
■ Deep-Water Jogging (fwd/retro): *5* min.
❏ Deep-Water Groin Stretch
❏ Knee to Chest Reps: ____
❏ Closed Kinematic Chain Exercises
❏ Deep-Water Double Knee Lifts Reps: ____
❏ Wall Slide Reps: ____
❏ Pelvic Tilts Reps: ____
❏ Supine Kicks Reps: ____
❏ Deep-Water Spinal Traction in Vertical Suspension
    (____ lbs. x ____ min.)
❏ Resistive Exercises:

■ Other: *Metered ambulation in shallow water with oximetry*

Aquatic Work Conditioning

❏ Resistive Forward/Retro Gait x ____ laps
❏ Deep-Water Jogging (fwd/retro) x ____ min.
❏ Tethered Jogging # ____ x ____ min.
❏ Swimming: ____ laps/min

❏ Other:

Equipment Used

■ Bodyfit® Collar
❏ Floatation Vest
❏ Tire Tube
■ Floatation Pelvic Belt
❏ Fins
■ Snorkel Mask
❏ Snorkel Tube
❏ Ankle Floats
❏ Aqua-Dumbbells

■ AquaJogger
❏ Graduated-Resistance Paddles
❏ Hydrotone Boots
❏ Hoola Hoop
❏ Resistance Cord
❏ Thera-Band®
❏ Aquakinetic Machines
❏ Boards
❏ Floatation Noodle

❏ Hydrotone Dumbbells
❏ Weights: ____
■ Bad Ragaz Floatation Rings
❏ Swim Bar
❏ Recumbent Bicycle
❏ Underwater Treadmill
■ Halliwick Blow Balls
❏ Other:

Adjunct Therapy

■ Not Applicable

❏ Whirlpool: ____ min. (spa)
❏ Patient Education
❏ Posture and Body Mechanics
❏ Home Exercise Program

❏ Other:

Land Based Therapy Treatments

■ Not Applicable

Frequency: ____ times per week
    for ____ weeks
❏ US: _____
❏ ES: _____
❏ HP's: _____
❏ Massage: _____

❏ Therapeutic Exercises (specify):
❏ Paraffin Bath:
❏ Cryotherapy:
❏ Joint Mobilization:
❏ Piriformis Release

Comments:

_____   _____
Signature & Credentials of Therapist   Date

Discussion

Based on the documented clinical findings, the interventions selected in the care plan for this case are aimed at improving chest excursions and strengthening the diaphragm and intercostal musculature through applied stretch reflex facilitation and improving vital capacity. Additional activities include those focusing on energy conservation and prevention of excessive fatigue even though the patient might progress to more physically complex activities. Although the patient with asthma presents clinical signs and symptoms that should be monitored, this type of patient tends to have a higher tolerance level than the patient with emphysema. This is reflected in the muscle strength results. Generally, this type of patient is also much more physically active than the patient with emphysema. Clinical manifestations must also be considered. If the patient is dyspneic, activities should be modified accordingly. Patients with asthma will generally not be oxygen dependent, but their bronchodilator must be kept available for use at all times.

Atelectasis

Atelectasis is a segmental, lobular, or total collapse of a lung caused externally (by compression) or internally (from an obstructed airway). The clinical assessment of the patient with atelectasis focuses on auscultation, thoracic symmetry, and mediate percussion. The primary problem is ventilation of the collapsed area. If the area is not ventilated adequately, proper perfusion cannot take place and this could consequently affect the diffusion capabilities. Atelectasis generally occurs as a clinical manifestation or result of the overall clinical picture or diagnosis.

Unless the cause of the collapse is airway obstruction by a lodged mucous plug, patients with atelectasis are "dry." Therefore, the therapist should place emphasis on improving ventilation to the area by strengthening the primary respiratory musculature and enhancing inspiratory effort. Reeducation of breathing patterns, improvement of inspiratory capacity, and improvement of tidal volume are the primary goals. Segmental breathing techniques should be integrated into selected Bad Ragaz patterns. The Bad Ragaz unilateral and bilateral upper extremity patterns could prove very effective in meeting the primary goals. Since Watsu® integrates the practice of breathing techniques, it is considered an effective intervention.

Furthermore, instructions and practice on the three phases of breathing control featured in the Clinical Wassertanzen Protocol will further improve widespread ventilation bilaterally. Patients should be able to master each phase before progressing to the next one. If the patient experiences fear of being submersed, the emphasis should remain on the first two phases. Another effective aquatic rehabilitation approach to the treatment of the patient with atelectasis is the integration of prone activity using mask and snorkel.

Atelectasis Case Study

The following case study uses the DASI pre-aquatic assessment form to present clinical findings, establish goals, and select the interventions that best meet the goals. A discussion of the case follows to justify the selection of activities, techniques, and interventions and to suggest other potentially effective strategies in the clinical management of the patient with atelectasis.

DASI
Diagnostic Aquatics Systems Integration — Pre-Aquatic Therapy Assessment

Patient Name: _____Steven_____   Date: _____

Dx: ___RLL Atelectasis_____   Age: ___32_____

History/Problems/Complaints: *Pt. sustained GSW to the right base of the chest. Chest tube inserted while admitted to the hospital. Post ICU hospital recovery lasted 10 days. Recurrent episodes of rt. basal collapse continue. Current CXR shows rt. elevated hemidiaphragm. PFT's demonstrate a decreased tidal volume and inspiratory capacity.*
Clinical Impression: *Ventilation-perfusion dysfunction; weak respiratory muscles*

Musculoskeletal Assessment

Musculoskeletal Assessment		Manual Muscle Test		Range of Motion	
		Right	Left	Right	Left
Shoulder	Flexors	5/5	5/5	WFL	WFL
	Extensors	5/5	5/5	WFL	WFL
	Abductors	5/5	5/5	WFL	WFL
	Adductors	5/5	5/5	WFL	WFL
	External Rotators	5/5	5/5	WFL	WFL
	Internal Rotators	5/5	5/5	WFL	WFL
Elbow	Flexors	5/5	5/5	WFL	WFL
	Extensors	5/5	5/5	WFL	WFL
Forearm	Pronators	5/5	5/5	WFL	WFL
	Supinators	5/5	5/5	WFL	WFL
Wrist	Flexors	5/5	5/5	WFL	WFL
	Extensors	5/5	5/5	WFL	WFL
Finger	Flexors/Hand Grip	5/5	5/5	WFL	WFL
Hip	Flexors	5/5	5/5	WFL	WFL
	Extensors	5/5	5/5	WFL	WFL
	Abductors	5/5	5/5	WFL	WFL
	Adductors	5/5	5/5	WFL	WFL
	External Rotators	5/5	5/5	WFL	WFL
	Internal Rotators	5/5	5/5	WFL	WFL

Musculoskeletal Assessment		Manual Muscle Test		Range of Motion	
		Right	Left	Right	Left
Knee	Flexors	5/5	5/5	WFL	WFL
	Extensors	5/5	5/5	WFL	WFL
Ankle	Dorsiflexors	5/5	5/5	WFL	WFL
	Plantar Flexors	5/5	5/5	WFL	WFL
Foot	Invertors	5/5	5/5	WFL	WFL
	Evertors	5/5	5/5	WFL	WFL

Musculoskeletal Assessment		ROM	MMT
Spine	Cervical Flexion	WFL	5/5
	Cervical Extension	WFL	5/5
	Cervical Lateral Flexion (right)	WFL	5/5
	Cervical Lateral Flexion (left)	WFL	5/5
	Cervical Rotation (right)	WFL	5/5
	Cervical Rotation (left)	WFL	5/5
	Lumbar Flexion	WFL	5/5
	Lumbar Extension	WFL	5/5
	Lumbar Lateral Flexion (right)	WFL	5/5
	Lumbar Lateral Flexion (left)	WFL	5/5

Evidence of Edema?   ❑ Yes   ■ No

Girth Anatomical Landmark: _____ ■ Not Applicable

Right:	_____inch(es)	Left:	_____ inch(es)

Leg-Length Discrepancy?   ❑ Yes   ■ No
Approximate Discrepancy: _____ inch(es)

Musculoskeletal Assessment (continued)

Posture

Posture		
	❏ Normal Alignment ■ Postural Deviations	**Explain** *Harrison's Groove Deformity*

Spasmodic Activity

	❏ No evidence of muscle spasms ❏ Not applicable	**Grade**			
		1	2	3	4
Spasmodic Activity	**Muscles**				
	rt SCM		■		
	lt SCM		■		

Cardiopulmonary Assessment

Cardiopulmonary Assessment

Lungs	❏ Clear to Auscultation ■ Abnormal Breath Sounds *Diminished breath sounds at RLL* ❏ Adventitious Breath Sounds ❏ Resonant Chest to Mediate Percussion ❏ Other: ■ Bibasilar Thoracic Asymmetry *Lt. > Rt.* RR: _____ ■ Normal ❏ Dyspnea ■ Other: *Bronchophony RLL*	
Cardiac	■ Normal S1 ■ Normal S2 ❏ Split S1 ❏ Split S2 ❏ S3 ❏ S4 ❏ Murmur ❏ Ejection Click HR: _____ BP: _____	Other:

Neurological Assessment

Neurologic Assessment

Superficial Sensation	■ Intact ❏ Impaired	**Explain**
Coordination	■ Intact ❏ Impaired ❏ Intention Tremors	**Explain**
Proprioception	■ Intact ❏ Impaired	**Explain**
Deep Tendon Reflexes	■ Intact ❏ Diminished _____ ❏ Hyperactive _____	**Explain**
Balance	Static ■ Intact ❏ Impaired Dynamic ■ Intact ❏ Impaired	

	No Pain								Intolerable Pain	
Pain	0	1	■	3	4	5	6	7 8	9	10

mild pain on inspiration at right base

Tone	■ Normal ❏ Hypertonia / Spasticity ❏ Hypotonia / Flaccidity ❏ Cogwheel Rigidity ❏ Contractures

	Check the Appropriate Box			
Other Neurologic Test Results		Pos	Neg	N/A
	SLR Test	❏	❏	■
	Neural Tension Ulnar Radial Median	❏	❏	■
	Fabere Sign	❏	❏	■
	Compression Test	❏	❏	■
	Distraction Stretch	❏	❏	■
	Vertebral Artery Test	❏	❏	■
	Alar Ligament Test	❏	❏	■
	Vertebral Glide Test	❏	❏	■
	Babinski Sign	❏	❏	■
	Romberg's Test	❏	❏	■
	Other	❏	❏	■

Functional Assessment

	Mobility
Gait Analysis	■ Ambulatory ❑ Non-Ambulatory Explain: ❑ Assistive Device: Weight Bearing: ■ FWB ❑ PWB ❑ NWB ❑ No significant gait deviations noted. ❑ Gait Deviations: ❑ Abnormal Gait
Bed Mobility	■ Independent ❑ Requires assistance ❑ max ❑ mod ❑ min
Transfers	■ Independent ❑ Requires assistance ❑ max ❑ mod ❑ min
Body Mechanics	■ Not tested ❑ Uses proper body mechanics when lifting, carrying, sitting, and lying down ❑ Does not use proper body mechanics when lifting, carrying, and lying down ❑ Needs further instruction and practice

Goals

■ Improve endurance
❑ Improve balance
❑ Improve spinal mobility
❑ Promote relaxation
■ Improve breathing patterns
Diaphragmatic, costolateral, segmental
■ Decrease pain
rt. base
❑ Increase muscle strength

❑ Increase joint range and flexibility

❑ Improve gait pattern
❑ Improve coordination and proprioception
❑ Reduce muscle fatigue
❑ Decrease edema and inflammation

❑ Improve postural alignment
❑ Improve circulation
❑ Improve motor control
❑ Inhibit spasticity/hypertonicity

❑ Resolution of muscle spasms:
SCM

Plan of Care

Frequency: __3__ times per week for __4__ weeks

Bad Ragaz	■ Passive Relaxation ❑ Passive Pelvic Tilts ❑ Pre-Gait ❑ Isotonic #1 ❑ Isotonic #2 ❑ Isometric ❑ Pre-Weight-Bearing ❑ Tone Inhibition ❑ Passive Trunk Elongation/Knee Hold ❑ Passive Trunk Elongation/Pelvic Hold ■ Passive Trunk Elongation/Thoracic Hold ■ Unilateral Upper Extremity ■ Bilateral Upper Extremity ■ Prone Unilateral Upper Extremity ■ Unilateral Lower Extremity ❑ Bilateral Lower Extremity ❑ Bilateral Symmetrical Lower Extremity #1 ❑ Bilateral Symmetrical Lower Extremity #2 ❑ Bilateral Reciprocal Lower Extremity ■ Other: *Passive trunk elongation w/ elbow hold*
Halliwick	❑ Phase I Adjustment ❑ Phase II Rotational Activities ❑ Turbulent Gliding ❑ Balance Training/Kangaroo Jumps ❑ Balance Training/Weight Shifting ■ Other: *Halliwick breathing activities with flip balls*

Cardiaquatics	❑ Level I Sequences: _____ Activities: _____
	❑ Level II Sequences: _____ Activities: _____
	❑ Level III Sequences: _____ Activities: _____
	❑ Level IV
	     ❑ Phase 1 ❑ Phase 2 ❑ Phase 3 ❑ All
	     ❑ Selected Sequences:

Other	❑ Applied Myofascial Release ❑ Deep Friction Massage ❑ Applied Joint Mobilization/Distraction ❑ Applied Spinal Mobilization/Distraction ❑ Applied Joint Approximation ❑ Applied Feldenkrais ❑ Applied Lymphatic Drainage ■ Watsu/Basic Flow ■ Watsu/Transitional Flow ■ Clinical Wassertanzen I ■ Clinical Wassertanzen II ❑ Clinical Wassertanzen III ❑ Applied Aquatic Craniosacral Therapy ❑ Trigger Point Therapy ■ Ai Chi: *Upper extremity exercises* ❑ Spinal/Trunk Stabilization Protocol: ❑ Thoracic Outlet Syndrome Protocol: ❑ Other: _____

Functional / Goal Specific Aquatic Therapy Activities and Exercises

- ■ Gait Training (Forward/Backward) Laps: *1-3*
- ❏ Stair Climbing x _____
- ❏ Bicycling Reps: _____
- ■ Prone Activities Min *3-5*
- ❏ Aquajogging Laps: _____
- ❏ Heal Cord Stretch
- ❏ Iliopsoas Stretch
- ❏ Piriformis Stretch
- ❏ TFL Stretch
- ❏ IT Band Stretch
- ❏ Hip Add Stretch
- ❏ Stork Stand
- ❏ Front to Back Weight Shifting
- ❏ Side to Side Weight Shifting
- ❏ Heel Raises Reps: _____
- ❏ Four-Corner Pivot Reps: _____

- ❏ Side-Stepping Laps: _____
- ❏ Cross Over Stepping Laps: _____
- ❏ Deep-Water Stride Jump Reps: _____
- ■ Deep-Water Jogging (fwd/retro): *5* min.
- ❏ Deep-Water Groin Stretch
- ❏ Knee to Chest Reps: _____
- ❏ Closed Kinematic Chain Exercises
- ❏ Deep-Water Double Knee Lifts Reps: _____
- ❏ Wall Slide Reps: _____
- ❏ Pelvic Tilts Reps: _____
- ❏ Supine Kicks Reps: _____
- ❏ Deep-Water Spinal Traction in Vertical Suspension
  (_____ lbs. x _____ min.)
- ❏ Resistive Exercises:

- ■ Other: *Metered ambulation in shallow water with oximetry*

Aquatic Work Conditioning

- ❏ Resistive Forward/Retro Gait x _____ laps
- ❏ Deep-Water Jogging (fwd/retro) x _____ min.
- ❏ Tethered Jogging # _____ x _____ min.
- ❏ Swimming: _____ laps/min

- ❏ Other: _____

Equipment Used

- ■ Bodyfit® Collar
- ❏ Floatation Vest
- ❏ Tire Tube
- ■ Floatation Pelvic Belt
- ❏ Fins
- ■ Snorkel Mask
- ■ Snorkel Tube
- ❏ Ankle Floats
- ❏ Aqua-Dumbbells

- ■ AquaJogger
- ❏ Graduated-Resistance Paddles
- ❏ Hydrotone Boots
- ❏ Hoola Hoop
- ❏ Resistance Cord
- ❏ Thera-Band®
- ❏ Aquakinetic Machines
- ❏ Boards
- ❏ Floatation Noodle

- ❏ Hydrotone Dumbbells
- ❏ Weights: _____
- ■ Bad Ragaz Floatation Rings
- ❏ Swim Bar
- ❏ Recumbent Bicycle
- ❏ Underwater Treadmill
- ■ Halliwick Blow Balls
- ❏ Other: _____

Adjunct Therapy

- ■ Not Applicable

- ❏ Whirlpool: _____ min. (spa)
- ❏ Patient Education
- ❏ Posture and Body Mechanics
- ❏ Home Exercise Program

- ❏ Other: _____

Land Based Therapy Treatments

- ■ Not Applicable

- Frequency: _____ times per week
  for _____ weeks
- ❏ US: _____
- ❏ ES: _____
- ❏ HP's: _____
- ❏ Massage: _____

- ❏ Therapeutic Exercises (specify):
- ❏ Paraffin Bath:
- ❏ Cryotherapy:
- ❏ Joint Mobilization:
- ❏ Piriformis Release

Comments:
Integrate segmental breathing in all shallow and deep-water activities. Measurement of the patient's inspiration rates should be taken before and after each aquatic session.

_____   _____

Signature & Credentials of Therapist   Date

Discussion

A patient with atelectasis might present with no deficits in muscle strength, range of motion, or girth. Nor might he present any evidence of neurological signs with the possible exception of pain. The source of pain depends on the primary diagnosis, e.g., if the collapse was caused by a gunshot wound that required chest tube insertion. The primary goal is to increase ventilation in the affected area. The interventions selected (Watsu, Wassertanzen, Halliwick in this case) are aimed at the main goal. All other integrated functional aquatic activities (shallow and deep-water dynamic activities) should also incorporate the practice of coordinated deep breathing exercises. Inspirometry would provide information on the patient's progress towards goal attainment.

Partially Rehabilitated and Cardiac Risk Factor

Phase IV cardiac rehabilitation is generally defined as an unsupervised program of physical activities that promote cardiovascular fitness. Even though my Cardiaquatics Protocol is considered a phase IV program, it requires supervision and monitoring by a credentialed and experienced aquatic rehabilitation therapist. As a requirement for admission into the Cardiaquatics Protocol, the patient should have completed phases I, II, and III cardiac rehabilitation. Additionally, a conference call between the aquatic therapist and the referring physician should be made to clarify any questions or issues surrounding the patient's medical history. The physician must be well informed about the structure of the protocol, including levels, sequences, and activities. The specific clinical goals should also be established. Once the physician understands the protocol, he can provide full clearance for the patient or identify limitations and precautions that apply to a particular patient. This allows the aquatic therapist to be prescriptive about the levels, sequences, and activities selected for the patient, making it a tailored protocol for each individual patient.

In order to arrive at a prescriptive decision, focusing on goals and plans of care, the therapist should complete a comprehensive pre-aquatic assessment using the DASI evaluation form. Documentation of the patient's history should include a list of medications (e.g., beta blockers, calcium channel blockers, vasodilators, antiarrhythmics, or cardiac glycosides) that the patient is taking at the time of the evaluation. In addition, the therapist should document whether or not the patient has undergone surgical intervention and, if so, specify the type of surgery that the patient had (e.g., coronary artery bypass graft, semilunar valvuloplasty or atrioventricular valvuloplasty). The cardiopulmonary assessment component of the evaluation should emphasize cardiac auscultation and a review of the results of the most recent graded exercise tolerance test (stress test).

Any risk factor history should also be documented. One of the most common risk factors is essential or systemic hypertension. Intensive monitoring of blood pressure and the effects of exercise in combination with antihypertensives must be the central focus of the plan of care. Another risk factor to consider is diabetes mellitus. Some literature has established that physical activity through exercises decreases and stabilizes glucose levels.

DASI
Diagnostic Aquatics Systems Integration — Pre-Aquatic Therapy Assessment

Patient Name: _____*Bob*_____   Date: _____

Dx: ___*Status Post Anterolateral MI*_____   Age: ___*48*_____

History/Problems/Complaints: *Pt. underwent cardiac rehab. Phases I, II and III at Memorial Hospital. His hospital recovery course was uncomplicated. Discharge medications include NTG prn, Inderal 80 mg LA, and Isordil 20 mg. Most recent GXTT using the Bruce Protocol was completed successfully and unremarkably without any indications of arrhythmic activity or onset of angina. Pt. was an avid tennis player prior to his cardiac event and has indicated his desire to resume his active lifestyle. The patient denies episodes of angina since his cardiac event. His risk factors include past smoking hx of 1 ppd currently controlled since he enrolled in a smoking cessation clinic, hypertension, and type A personality. The patient is currently employed as an executive vice-president at a major corporation.*
Clinical Impression: *Decreased cardiovascular endurance*

Musculoskeletal Assessment

Musculoskeletal Assessment		Manual Muscle Test		Range of Motion	
		Right	Left	Right	Left
Shoulder	Flexors	5/5	5/5	WFL	WFL
	Extensors	5/5	5/5	WFL	WFL
	Abductors	5/5	5/5	WFL	WFL
	Adductors	5/5	5/5	WFL	WFL
	External Rotators	5/5	5/5	WFL	WFL
	Internal Rotators	5/5	5/5	WFL	WFL
Elbow	Flexors	5/5	5/5	WFL	WFL
	Extensors	5/5	5/5	WFL	WFL
Forearm	Pronators	5/5	5/5	WFL	WFL
	Supinators	5/5	5/5	WFL	WFL
Wrist	Flexors	5/5	5/5	WFL	WFL
	Extensors	5/5	5/5	WFL	WFL
Finger	Flexors/Hand Grip	5/5	5/5	WFL	WFL
Hip	Flexors	5/5	5/5	WFL	WFL
	Extensors	5/5	5/5	WFL	WFL
	Abductors	5/5	5/5	WFL	WFL
	Adductors	5/5	5/5	WFL	WFL
	External Rotators	5/5	5/5	WFL	WFL
	Internal Rotators	5/5	5/5	WFL	WFL

Musculoskeletal Assessment		Manual Muscle Test		Range of Motion	
		Right	Left	Right	Left
Knee	Flexors	5/5	5/5	WFL	WFL
	Extensors	5/5	5/5	WFL	WFL
Ankle	Dorsiflexors	5/5	5/5	WFL	WFL
	Plantar Flexors	5/5	5/5	WFL	WFL
Foot	Invertors	5/5	5/5	WFL	WFL
	Evertors	5/5	5/5	WFL	WFL

Musculoskeletal Assessment		ROM	MMT
Spine	Cervical Flexion	WFL	5/5
	Cervical Extension	WFL	5/5
	Cervical Lateral Flexion (right)	WFL	5/5
	Cervical Lateral Flexion (left)	WFL	5/5
	Cervical Rotation (right)	WFL	5/5
	Cervical Rotation (left)	WFL	5/5
	Lumbar Flexion	WFL	5/5
	Lumbar Extension	WFL	5/5
	Lumbar Lateral Flexion (right)	WFL	5/5
	Lumbar Lateral Flexion (left)	WFL	5/5

Evidence of Edema?   ❏ Yes   ■ No

Leg-Length Discrepancy?   ❏ Yes   ■ No
Approximate Discrepancy: _____ inch(es)

Girth Anatomical Landmark: ____ ■ Not Applicable

Right:	_____ inch(es)	Left:	_____ inch(es)

Cardiopulmonary Assessment

Musculoskeletal Assessment (continued)

Posture

	□ Normal Alignment ■ Postural Deviations Explain: *anteriorly rotated pelvis with some degree of lordosis*

Posture (left vertical label)

Spasmodic Activity				
□ No evidence of muscle spasms □ Not applicable	**Grade**			
	1	2	3	4

Muscles				
spinalis		■		
longissimus		■		
rt. piriformis		■		
bilat. upper traps		■		

Spasmodic Activity (left vertical label)

Cardiopulmonary Assessment

Lungs

- ■ Clear to Auscultation
- □ Abnormal Breath Sounds
- □ Adventitious Breath Sounds
- □ Resonant Chest to Mediate Percussion
- □ Other:
- □ Bibasilar Thoracic Asymmetry

RR: _____ ■ Normal □ Dyspnea □ Other:

Cardiac

	Other:
■ Normal S1 ■ Normal S2 □ Split S1 □ Split S2 □ S3 ■ S4 □ Murmur □ Ejection Click HR: *82* BP: *138/84*	

Neurological Assessment

Neurologic Assessment	
Superficial Sensation ■ Intact □ Impaired	**Explain**
Coordination ■ Intact □ Impaired □ Intention Tremors	**Explain**
Proprioception ■ Intact □ Impaired	**Explain**
Deep Tendon Reflexes ■ Intact □ Diminished _____ □ Hyperactive _____	**Explain**
Balance Static ■ Intact □ Impaired Dynamic ■ Intact □ Impaired	

Pain

No Pain								Intolerable Pain
■ 1	2	3	4	5	6	7	8	9 10

Tone

- ■ Normal
- □ Hypertonia / Spasticity
- □ Hypotonia / Flaccidity
- □ Cogwheel Rigidity
- □ Contractures

Other Neurologic Test Results

	Check the Appropriate Box		
	Pos	Neg	N/A
SLR Test	□	□	■
Neural Tension	□	□	■
Ulnar Radial Median			
Fabere Sign	□	□	■
Compression Test	□	□	■
Distraction Stretch	□	□	■
Vertebral Artery Test	□	□	■
Alar Ligament Test	□	□	■
Vertebral Glide Test	□	□	■
Babinski Sign	□	□	■
Romberg's Test	□	□	■
Other	□	□	■

Functional Assessment

	Mobility
Gait Analysis	■ Ambulatory ❏ Non-Ambulatory Explain: ❏ Assistive Device: Weight Bearing: ■ FWB ❏ PWB ❏ NWB ■ No significant gait deviations noted. ❏ Gait Deviations: ❏ Abnormal Gait
Bed Mobility	■ Independent ❏ Requires assistance ❏ max ❏ mod ❏ min
Transfers	■ Independent ❏ Requires assistance ❏ max ❏ mod ❏ min
Body Mechanics	❏ Not tested ❏ Uses proper body mechanics when lifting, carrying, sitting, and lying down ■ Does not use proper body mechanics when lifting, carrying, and lying down ■ Needs further instruction and practice

Goals

■ Improve endurance
❏ Improve balance
❏ Improve spinal mobility
■ Promote relaxation
■ Improve breathing patterns
maintain adequate tidal volume and vital capacity
❏ Decrease pain

_____

❏ Increase muscle strength

_____

❏ Increase joint range and flexibility

_____

❏ Improve gait pattern
❏ Improve coordination and proprioception
❏ Reduce muscle fatigue
❏ Decrease edema and inflammation

_____

❏ Improve postural alignment
❏ Improve circulation
❏ Improve motor control
❏ Inhibit spasticity/hypertonicity

_____

■ Resolution of muscle spasms:
as identified in the spasmodic activity evaluation

Plan of Care

Frequency: _____ times per week for _____ weeks

Bad Ragaz	■ Passive Relaxation ❏ Passive Pelvic Tilts ❏ Pre-Gait ❏ Isotonic #1 ❏ Isotonic #2 ❏ Isometric ❏ Pre-Weight-Bearing ❏ Tone Inhibition ❏ Passive Trunk Elongation/Knee Hold ❏ Passive Trunk Elongation/Pelvic Hold ❏ Passive Trunk Elongation/Thoracic Hold ❏ Unilateral Upper Extremity ❏ Bilateral Upper Extremity ❏ Prone Unilateral Upper Extremity ❏ Unilateral Lower Extremity ❏ Bilateral Lower Extremity ❏ Bilateral Symmetrical Lower Extremity #1 ❏ Bilateral Symmetrical Lower Extremity #2 ❏ Bilateral Reciprocal Lower Extremity ❏ Other:
Halliwick	❏ Phase I Adjustment ❏ Phase II Rotational Activities ❏ Turbulent Gliding ❏ Balance Training/Kangaroo Jumps ❏ Balance Training/Weight Shifting ❏ Other: _____
Cardiaquatics	■ Level I Sequences: *All* Activities: *All* ■ Level II Sequences: *All* Activities: *All* ■ Level III Sequences: *All* Activities: *All* ■ Level IV 　■ Phase 1 ❏ Phase 2 ■ Phase 3 ❏ All 　❏ Selected Sequences:
Other	❏ Applied Myofascial Release ❏ Deep Friction Massage ❏ Applied Joint Mobilization/Distraction ❏ Applied Spinal Mobilization/Distraction ❏ Applied Joint Approximation ❏ Applied Feldenkrais ❏ Applied Lymphatic Drainage ■ Watsu/Basic Flow ■ Watsu/Transitional Flow ■ Clinical Wassertanzen I ■ Clinical Wassertanzen II ■ Clinical Wassertanzen III ❏ Applied Aquatic Craniosacral Therapy ■ Trigger Point Therapy ■ Ai Chi: *upper extremity exercises* ❏ Spinal/Trunk Stabilization Protocol: ❏ Thoracic Outlet Syndrome Protocol: ❏ Other: _____

Functional / Goal Specific Aquatic Therapy Activities and Exercises

❐ Gait Training (Forward/Backward) Laps: _____
❐ Stair Climbing x _____
❐ Bicycling Reps: _____
❐ Prone Activities Min _____
❐ Aquajogging Laps: _____
■ Heal Cord Stretch
■ Iliopsoas Stretch
■ Piriformis Stretch
■ TFL Stretch
■ IT Band Stretch
■ Hip Add Stretch
❐ Stork Stand
❐ Front to Back Weight Shifting
❐ Side to Side Weight Shifting
❐ Heel Raises Reps: _____
❐ Four-Corner Pivot Reps: _____

❐ Side-Stepping Laps: _____
❐ Cross Over Stepping Laps: _____
❐ Deep-Water Stride Jump Reps: _____
❐ Deep-Water Jogging (fwd/retro): _____ min.
❐ Deep-Water Groin Stretch
❐ Knee to Chest Reps: _____
❐ Closed Kinematic Chain Exercises
❐ Deep-Water Double Knee Lifts Reps: _____
❐ Wall Slide Reps: _____
❐ Pelvic Tilts Reps: _____
❐ Supine Kicks Reps:_____
❐ Deep-Water Spinal Traction in Vertical Suspension
(_____ lbs. x _____ min.)
❐ Resistive Exercises:

❐ Other:_____

Aquatic Work Conditioning

❐ Resistive Forward/Retro Gait x _____ laps
❐ Deep-Water Jogging (fwd/retro) x _____ min.
■ Tethered Jogging # *5* x *1* min.
❐ Swimming: _____laps/min

❐ Other:_____

Equipment Used

■ Bodyfit® Collar
❐ Floatation Vest
❐ Tire Tube
❐ Floatation Pelvic Belt
❐ Fins
■ Snorkel Mask
■ Snorkel Tube
❐ Ankle Floats
■ Aqua-Dumbbells

■ AquaJogger
■ Graduated-Resistance Paddles
❐ Hydrotone Boots
❐ Hoola Hoop
❐ Resistance Cord
❐ Thera-Band®
❐ Aquakinetic Machines
❐ Boards
❐ Floatation Noodle

❐ Hydrotone Dumbbells
❐ Weights: _____
■ Bad Ragaz Floatation Rings
❐ Swim Bar
❐ Recumbent Bicycle
❐ Underwater Treadmill
❐ Halliwick Blow Balls
❐ Other:_____

Adjunct Therapy

■ Not Applicable

❐ Whirlpool: _____ min. (spa)
❐ Patient Education
❐ Posture and Body Mechanics
❐ Home Exercise Program

❐ Other:_____

Land Based Therapy Treatments

■ Not Applicable

Frequency: _____ times per week
for _____ weeks
❐ US: _____
❐ ES: _____
❐ HP's: _____
❐ Massage: _____

❐ Therapeutic Exercises (specify):
❐ Paraffin Bath:
❐ Cryotherapy:
❐ Joint Mobilization:
❐ Piriformis Release

Comments: *Full Cardiaquatics protocol with the integration of selected aquatic work-conditioning activities as identified. Monitor BP and HR as requested and required in the protocol. Flow basic guidelines for progression and contraindication of activities. Integrated Wassertanzen will maintain adequate respiratory dynamics. Passive and active stretches to be emphasized to elongate shortened structures in preparation for activities.*

_____   _____
Signature & Credentials of Therapist   Date

Discussion

This type of patient is the ideal candidate for a full protocol. However, if the patient's recovery course has been complicated, the protocol can be tailored to the patient and the activities may be modified according to the patient's condition and tolerance. In this example, all levels, sequences, and activities will be practiced. However, these should be gradually and progressively integrated into the plan of care as opposed to practicing the full protocol in one session. This will ascertain tolerance and progressively acquired endurance, which is one of the primary goals. Instruction and practice on active stretches must be integrated in the pre-activity preparatory phase. These stretches should concentrate on the elongation of structures that influence the identified postural deficits such as the anteriorly rotated pelvis. These feature the hip flexors. Additionally, manual trigger point releases to the piriformis muscle should be applied before and after the Cardiaquatics protocol session in an effort to improve posture and prevent low back and hip pain associated with a possible development of piriformis syndrome. This case integrates interventions that are aimed at enhancing cardiovascular fitness and endurance, and includes prevention techniques as well.

CHAPTER 10

INTEGRATED NEUROLOGY

Parkinson's Disease

Parkinson's disease is a disorder of the basal ganglia affecting primarily the substantia nigra. Patients who are diagnosed with Parkinson's disease exhibit prototypical clinical manifestations that include, but are not limited to, cogwheel rigidity, intention tremors, and a festinating gait. There are problems with voluntary activity that reflect in akinesia (difficulty initiating movement) or bradykinesia (a slow movement pattern with difficulty in controlling movement). However, the patients with Parkinson's disease can also have involuntary movement disorders that influence the degree of rigidity and the incidence of tremors. Although the etiology of Parkinson's disease remains largely idiopathic, it has been established that causes can include exposure to toxins, infections, trauma, and hereditary factors.

One of the significant motor problems exhibited by the patient with Parkinson's disease is the presence of abnormally increased tone. When the therapist attempts to passively move an extremity or joint through its normal range, he will feel involuntary jerky motions throughout the full range. This is referred to as cogwheel rigidity and is characteristic of the type of spasticity present in the patient with Parkinson's disease. Even if the condition is not advanced and cogwheel rigidity is not yet an impediment to motor activity, the patient will tend to exhibit some degree of generalized hypertonicity.

The incidence of intention tremors is also a prototypical manifestation of the patient with Parkinson's disease. In addition to the motor deficits reflected in the clinical manifestations, the tremors affect coordination and proprioception as well. An intention tremor occurs primarily when the patient attempts to perform a purposeful activity. It is described as a rapid shaking of the extremity with phasic involuntary contractions of agonists and antagonists alike. In addition, 70% of patients with Parkinson's disease also tend to exhibit involuntary rhythmic resting tremors.

Patients with Parkinson's disease walk with short strides, decreased cadence, and shuffling, fast, uncoordinated steps. This is referred to as a festinating gait and occurs as a result of the rigidity, hypertonicity, and poor coordination that characterize the disease. Initiating gait is difficult, but even more difficult is controlling the speed and cadence of the gait pattern once the activity is initiated. These clinical problems also reflect in postural malalignment.

Pharmacotherapy has been successful in prolonging remission in the patient with Parkinson's disease. The objective of pharmacotherapy is to alleviate the clinical manifestations that interfere with the patient's day-to-day functions. Land-based therapy has also proven effective in the attainment of functional outcomes and goals for these patients. Spasticity inhibiting techniques are commonly used along with activities to promote coordination. However, it is important to consider that these patients tend to experience a "roller-coaster effect," that is, their improvement plateaus for a limited period of time and then the clinical manifestations recur.

Aquatic rehabilitation is one of the new approaches in the clinical management of the patient with Parkinson's disease. I noticed that when treating these patients with selected aquatic therapy interventions they experienced a decrease in tone, an improvement in gait pattern, and an improvement in coordination. The application of Watsu® for these patients has been particularly effective in achieving the noted changes. However, further research is necessary to validate these outcomes.

The Bad Ragaz tone inhibition pattern can help to initially decrease hypertonia and prepare the patient for the Watsu® session. Other Bad Ragaz patterns that could complement the plan of care include the bilateral symmetrical lower extremity #1 and #2. These must be applied without resistance. Applying the bilateral repetitive lower extremity flexor patterns that characteristically initiate the Watsu® session may be a challenge for the therapist, particularly if the patient presents with significant extensor spasticity. Therefore, the integration of techniques that promote relaxation, such as the Bad Ragaz passive relaxation position, is highly advised. The Bad Ragaz bilateral and unilateral upper extremity patterns will affect coordination and kinesthesia.

Parkinson's Case Study

The following case utilizes the DASI pre-aquatic assessment form to present clinical findings, establish goals, and select interventions that would best meet the established goals. A discussion of the case is provided to justify the selection of activities, techniques, and interventions and to suggest other potentially effective strategies in the clinical management of the patient with Parkinson's disease.

DASI
Diagnostic Aquatics Systems Integration — Pre-Aquatic Therapy Assessment

Patient Name: _____*Andy*_____   Date: _____

Dx: __*Parkinson's disease*__   Age: ___*68*___

History/Problems/Complaints: *Pt. has a two-year h/o Parkinson's disease controlled by medication therapy. He exhibits mild dysarthria although he can articulate words and sentences, and is able to understand verbal commands. He was cooperative throughout the evaluation and treatment. His wife served as the source of information and interpreter.*

Clinical Impression: *Moderate to severe hypertonicity with gait, motor, and coordination deficits*

Musculoskeletal Assessment

Musculoskeletal Assessment		Manual Muscle Test		Range of Motion	
		Right	Left	Right	Left
Shoulder	Flexors	4/5	4/5	140°	145°
	Extensors	4/5	4/5	WFL	WFL
	Abductors	4/5	4/5	150°	140°
	Adductors	4/5	4/5	WFL	WFL
	External Rotators	4/5	4/5	40°	45°
	Internal Rotators	4/5	4/5	WFL	WFL
Elbow	Flexors	4/5	4/5	WFL	WFL
	Extensors	3/5	3/5	-20°	-20°
Forearm	Pronators	4/5	4/5	WFL	WFL
	Supinators	4/5	4/5	WFL	WFL
Wrist	Flexors	4/5	4/5	WFL	WFL
	Extensors	3-/5	3-/5	-90°	-90°
Finger	Flexors/Hand Grip	3/5	3/5	WFL	WFL
Hip	Flexors	3/5	3/5	WFL	WFL
	Extensors	4/5	4/5	-10°	-10°
	Abductors	3/5	3/5	WFL	WFL
	Adductors	4/5	4/5	WFL	WFL
	External Rotators	3/5	3/5	WFL	WFL
	Internal Rotators	3/5	3/5	WFL	WFL

Musculoskeletal Assessment		Manual Muscle Test		Range of Motion	
		Right	Left	Right	Left
Knee	Flexors	3/5	3/5	WFL	WFL
	Extensors	4/5	4/5	WFL	WFL
Ankle	Dorsiflexors	3/5	3/5	WFL	WFL
	Plantar Flexors	4/5	4/5	WFL	WFL
Foot	Invertors	4-/5	4-/5	WFL	WFL
	Evertors	4-/5	4-/5	WFL	WFL

Musculoskeletal Assessment	ROM	MMT
Spine Cervical Flexion	WFL	3+/5
Cervical Extension	-55°	3/5
Cervical Lateral Flexion (right)	5°	4/5
Cervical Lateral Flexion (left)	5°	4/5
Cervical Rotation (right)	5°	4/5
Cervical Rotation (left)	5°	4/5
Lumbar Flexion	20°	4-/5
Lumbar Extension	10°	4-/5
Lumbar Lateral Flexion (right)	10°	4-/5
Lumbar Lateral Flexion (left)	10°	4-/5

Evidence of Edema? ☐ Yes ■ No

Girth Anatomical Landmark: ____ ■ Not Applicable		
Right:	_____inch(es)	Left:	_____ inch(es)

Leg-Length Discrepancy? ☐ Yes ■ No
Approximate Discrepancy: _____ inch(es)

Musculoskeletal Assessment (continued)

Posture

Posture	
	❑ Normal Alignment
	■ Postural Deviations
	Explain *Forward head, forward shift, post. rotated pelvis, round shoulders*

Spasmodic Activity

		Grade			
❑ No evidence of muscle spasms					
■ Not applicable		1	2	3	4
Muscles					

Cardiopulmonary Assessment

Cardiopulmonary Assessment

Lungs

■ Clear to Auscultation
❑ Abnormal Breath Sounds

❑ Adventitious Breath Sounds

❑ Resonant Chest to Mediate Percussion
❑ Other:
■ Bibasilar Thoracic Asymmetry
Decreased bibasilar; increased biapical

RR: _____ ❑ Normal ❑ Dyspnea ❑ Other:

Cardiac

❑ Normal S1	Other:
■ Normal S2	
■ Split S1	
❑ Split S2	
❑ S3	
❑ S4	
❑ Murmur	
❑ Ejection Click	

HR: _____
BP: _____

Neurological Assessment

Neurologic Assessment

Superficial Sensation

■ Intact	**Explain**
❑ Impaired	

Coordination

❑ Intact   **Explain**
■ Impaired
■ Intention Tremors
Deficits noted in bilateral. upper and lower extremities

Proprioception

❑ Intact   **Explain**
■ Impaired
Impaired kinesthesia in both upper and lower extremities

Deep Tendon Reflexes

❑ Intact   **Explain**

❑ Diminished _____

■ Hyperactive *patellar and biceps bilaterally*

Balance

Static   ❑ Intact   ■ Impaired
Dynamic   ❑ Intact   ■ Impaired

Pain

No Pain   Intolerable Pain
■ 1   2   3   4   5   6   7   8   9   10

Tone

❑ Normal
■ Hypertonia / Spasticity
Extensor tone in LE's; flexor tone in UE's
❑ Hypotonia / Flaccidity
■ Cogwheel Rigidity
BUE's and BLE's
❑ Contractures

Other Neurologic Test Results

	Pos	Neg	N/A
SLR Test	❑	❑	■
Neural Tension	❑	❑	■
	Ulnar	Radial	Median
Fabere Sign	❑	❑	■
Compression Test	❑	❑	■
Distraction Stretch	❑	❑	■
Vertebral Artery Test	❑	❑	■
Alar Ligament Test	❑	❑	■
Vertebral Glide Test	❑	❑	■
Babinski Sign	❑	❑	■
Romberg's Test	❑	❑	
Other *bilateral clonus*	■	❑	❑

Functional Assessment

	Mobility
Gait Analysis	■ Ambulatory ❑Non-Ambulatory Explain: ❑ Assistive Device: Weight Bearing: ■ FWB ❑ PWB ❑ NWB ❑ No significant gait deviations noted. ■ Gait Deviations: *evid. of festinating gait* ■ Abnormal Gait *Bilateral shuffle w/decreased ankle dorsiflexion*
Bed Mobility	■ Independent ❑ Requires assistance ❑ max ❑ mod ❑ min
Transfers	■ Independent ❑ Requires assistance ❑ max ❑ mod ❑ min
Body Mechanics	■ Not tested ❑ Uses proper body mechanics when lifting, carrying, sitting, and lying down ❑ Does not use proper body mechanics when lifting, carrying, and lying down ❑ Needs further instruction and practice

Goals

■ Improve endurance
■ Improve balance
❑ Improve spinal mobility
■ Promote relaxation
■ Improve breathing patterns
Diaphragmatic and costolateral
❑ Decrease pain

❑ Increase muscle strength

❑ Increase joint range and flexibility

■ Improve gait pattern
■ Improve coordination and proprioception
❑ Reduce muscle fatigue
❑ Decrease edema and inflammation

■ Improve postural alignment
❑ Improve circulation
■ Improve motor control
■ Inhibit spasticity/hypertonicity
Extensor tone in BLE's and flexor tone in BUE's
❑ Resolution of muscle spasms:

Plan of Care

Frequency: _3_ times per week for _4_ weeks

Bad Ragaz	■ Passive Relaxation ❑ Passive Pelvic Tilts ❑ Pre-Gait ❑ Isotonic #1 ❑ Isotonic #2 ❑ Isometric ❑ Pre-Weight-Bearing ■ Tone Inhibition ❑ Passive Trunk Elongation/Knee Hold ❑ Passive Trunk Elongation/Pelvic Hold ■ Passive Trunk Elongation/Thoracic Hold ■ Unilateral Upper Extremity ■ Bilateral Upper Extremity ❑ Prone Unilateral Upper Extremity ❑ Unilateral Lower Extremity ❑ Bilateral Lower Extremity ■ Bilateral Symmetrical Lower Extremity #1 ❑ Bilateral Symmetrical Lower Extremity #2 ❑ Bilateral Reciprocal Lower Extremity ❑ Other: _____
Halliwick	❑ Phase I Adjustment ❑ Phase II Rotational Activities ❑ Turbulent Gliding ❑ Balance Training/Kangaroo Jumps ■ Balance Training/Weight Shifting ❑ Other: _____

Cardiaquatics	❑ Level I Sequences: ___ Activities: ___
	❑ Level II Sequences: ___ Activities: ___
	❑ Level III Sequences: ___ Activities: ___
	❑ Level IV
	  ❑ Phase 1 ❑ Phase 2 ❑ Phase 3 ❑ All
	  ❑ Selected Sequences:

Other	❑ Applied Myofascial Release ❑ Deep Friction Massage ❑ Applied Joint Mobilization/Distraction ❑ Applied Spinal Mobilization/Distraction ❑ Applied Joint Approximation ❑ Applied Feldenkrais ❑ Applied Lymphatic Drainage ■ Watsu/Basic Flow ■ Watsu/Transitional Flow ❑ Clinical Wassertanzen I ❑ Clinical Wassertanzen II ❑ Clinical Wassertanzen III ❑ Applied Aquatic Craniosacral Therapy ❑ Trigger Point Therapy ❑ Ai Chi: _____ ❑ Spinal/Trunk Stabilization Protocol: _____ ❑ Thoracic Outlet Syndrome Protocol: _____ ❑ Other: _____

Functional / Goal Specific Aquatic Therapy Activities and Exercises

■ Gait Training (<u>Forward/Backward</u>) Laps: *3*
❏ Stair Climbing x _____
❏ Bicycling Reps: _____
❏ Prone Activities Min _____
❏ Aquajogging Laps: _____
❏ Heel Cord Stretch
❏ Iliopsoas Stretch
❏ Piriformis Stretch
❏ TFL Stretch
❏ IT Band Stretch
❏ Hip Add Stretch
❏ Stork Stand
❏ Front to Back Weight Shifting
❏ Side to Side Weight Shifting
❏ Heel Raises Reps: _____
■ Four-Corner Pivot Reps: *3*

■ Side-Stepping Laps: *3*
❏ Cross Over Stepping Laps: _____
❏ Deep-Water Stride Jump Reps: _____
❏ Deep-Water Jogging (fwd/retro): _____ min.
❏ Deep-Water Groin Stretch
❏ Knee to Chest Reps: _____
❏ Closed Kinematic Chain Exercises
❏ Deep-Water Double Knee Lifts Reps: _____
❏ Wall Slide Reps: _____
❏ Pelvic Tilts Reps: ___
❏ Supine Kicks Reps:_____
❏ Deep-Water Spinal Traction in Vertical Suspension
  (_____ lbs. x _____ min.)
❏ Resistive Exercises:

■ Other: *Side-Stepping Crab Walk- 3 lbs fwd & bckwd*

Aquatic Work Conditioning

❏ Resistive Forward/Retro Gait x _____ laps
❏ Deep-Water Jogging (fwd/retro) x _____ min.
❏ Tethered Jogging # _____ x _____ min.
❏ Swimming: _____laps/min

❏ Other:_____

Equipment Used

■ Bodyfit® Collar
❏ Floatation Vest
❏ Tire Tube
■ Floatation Pelvic Belt
❏ Fins
❏ Snorkel Mask
❏ Snorkel Tube
❏ Ankle Floats
❏ Aqua-Dumbbells

❏ AquaJogger
❏ Graduated-Resistance Paddles
❏ Hydrotone Boots
❏ Hoola Hoop
❏ Resistance Cord
❏ Thera-Band®
❏ Aquakinetic Machines
❏ Boards
❏ Floatation Noodle

❏ Hydrotone Dumbbells
❏ Weights: _____
■ Bad Ragaz Floatation Rings
❏ Swim Bar
❏ Recumbent Bicycle
❏ Underwater Treadmill
❏ Halliwick Blow Balls
❏ Other:_____

Adjunct Therapy

■ Not Applicable

❏ Whirlpool: _____ min. (spa)
❏ Patient Education
❏ Posture and Body Mechanics
❏ Home Exercise Program

❏ Other:_____

Land Based Therapy Treatments

❏ Not Applicable

Frequency: _____ times per week
  for _____ weeks
❏ US: _____
❏ ES: _____
❏ HP's: _____
❏ Massage: _____

❏ Therapeutic Exercises (specify):
❏ Paraffin Bath:
■ Cryotherapy:
❏ Joint Mobilization:
❏ Piriformis Release

Ice massage to elbow and wrist flexor, hip and knee extensors, ankle plantar flexors
Comments:

_____   _____
Signature & Credentials of Therapist   Date

Discussion

The limitations in range of motion exhibited in this case follow the pattern of flexor spasticity in the upper extremities and extensor spasticity in the lower extremities particularly because the patient presents with a certain degree of cogwheel rigidity. Active range will be affected but a resistance to passive range will be felt. Limitations in spine range are consistent with postural deficits. The expected neurological tests will show impairment or abnormalities as stated. The postural deviation at the thorax might reflect a hollow chest deformity, which will tend to reveal decreased excursions at the bases and increases apically. Integration of interventions and techniques that promote relaxation are of utmost importance before any dynamic activity is practiced. The Bad Ragaz patterns selected are aimed at inhibiting spasticity, improving coordination and kinesthesia, and improving lateral costal and basal chest excursions.

Improving gait, coordination, and dynamic balance are the goals for which the dynamic shallow-water activities were selected. However, once these goals are achieved, other activities may be integrated, or the activities that are practiced may be made more challenging for the patient.

The cryotherapeutic application of ice to the hypertonic muscle groups will assist in diminishing tone and will decrease the degree of difficulty encountered by the therapist in the passive application of other interventions or by the patient as he practices the dynamic activities selected.

Traumatic Brain Injury

Rehabilitating the patient who has sustained a traumatic brain injury (TBI) presents a challenge for the therapist because we are not only dealing with sensory-motor deficits but with emotional, behavioral, and cognitive deficits as well. The psychological considerations have an effect on the patient, his family, and the attending therapist. Therefore, clinicians treating patients who have sustained a traumatic brain injury must have a global understanding of the social, psychological, and pathophysiological factors affecting the patient with a craniocerebral injury.

The etiology of injuries resulting from craniocerebral trauma is quite extensive but can be classified in two groups:

1. penetrating or open (e.g., gunshot wounds)
2. nonpenetrating or closed (e.g., impact injury from an automobile accident)

The extent and consequences of the injury will depend on the integrity of the dura mater, that is, whether or not there is bruising, tearing, or rupture (coup/countercoup) at the time of injury. Following an impact injury, lacerations and contusions of the underlying brain tissue can develop as a direct result of the impact and may be accompanied by skull fractures. These occur secondary to the rupture of arteries and veins that supply the underlying skull, meningeal, and brain tissue. Rupture of these vessels further leads to intracranial hemorrhage, which is manifested in the development of a subdural or epidural hematoma.

Brain damage can be classified as primary or secondary. Primary brain damage follows focal brain lesions while secondary brain damage is the result of systemically originated insults to the brain (e.g., hypoxemia, hypoglycemia). Common clinical manifestations include spasticity, decerebrate rigidity, decorticate rigidity, hypotonicity or flaccid paralysis, areflexia or dysreflexia, and hemiparesis or quadriparesis.

Decerebrate rigidity presents a clinical picture of severe extensor spasticity in both upper and lower extremities accompanied by arching with extension of the spine and neck. When there is evidence of decorticate rigidity, the patient presents the classic clinical picture of a flexor spastic pattern in the upper extremities with extensor spasticity in the lower extremities. Spasticity is a term used to define any abnormal increase in tone. The term "rigidity" designates a degree of advanced or severe spasticity that may precede the onset of contractures.

The patient who has sustained a TBI can benefit from selected aquatic rehabilitation interventions. The most important goal is to prevent the development of contractures, not only in the acute stages but subsequently as well. Later, during the rehabilitation phase, aquatic therapy can be integrated into the plan of care as other goals are considered.

If inhibition of tone figures among the clinical objectives, selected passive Bad Ragaz patterns can be performed, such as the tone inhibition pattern or a modified passive bilateral symmetrical lower extremity #1 pattern. Additionally, the Watsu® basic and transitional flow sequences could prove very effective in the inhibition of tone and decrease of rigidity. The same is true if the goal is to improve coordination or to begin gait training if the extent of the TBI is not severe. The Halliwick Method offers selected techniques that can assist in the improvement of balance, coordination, proprioception, and gait, particularly if ataxia is present. Ideally, Halliwick discourages the use of floatation devices. However, if there is a great deal of unsteadiness and safety is an issue, the therapist might consider using a floatation collar or floatation pelvic belt as needed.

Aquatic therapy should be supplemented with land therapy sessions. Patients with TBI are often apraxic and have difficulty with motor planning. Therefore, they will require an interdisciplinary approach to treatment involving all the members of the rehabilitation team on land and in the water.

If there is evidence of contractures, specially fabricated splints may be applied for use in the pool.

Depending on the degree and severity of the TBI, once initial goals are attained, other more dynamic aquatic therapy activities may be integrated into the aquatic rehabilitation plan of care emphasizing gait, posture, coordination, and muscle strength.

Traumatic Brain Injury Case Study

The following case utilizes the DASI pre-aquatic assessment form to present clinical findings, establish goals, and select the interventions that would best meet the established goals. A discussion of the case is provided to justify the selection of activities, techniques, and interventions and to suggest other potentially effective strategies in the clinical management of the patient who has sustained a traumatic brain injury.

DASI
Diagnostic Aquatics Systems Integration — Pre-Aquatic Therapy Assessment

Patient Name: _____Billy_____   Date: _____

Dx: ___TBI secondary to motor vehicle accident_____   Age: ___22_____

History/Problems/Complaints: *Billy was involved in an automobile accident one year ago, which left him in a coma for 3 months. After the accident he was admitted to the ICU, intubated, and placed on mechanical ventilation due to respiratory problems until he was tracheostomized one week later. He remained on mechanical ventilation via the Shiley tracheostomy tube for approximately one month at which time he showed improvement in his arterial blood gases. He then was placed on a nebulized oxygen source. As a result of injury to the motor cortex, Billy was rendered with decorticate rigidity. He exhibits receptive and expressive aphasia and apraxia. Consequently, the tests featured in the musculoskeletal assessment except for ROM were not performed. NT=not tested.*
Clinical Impression: *Decorticate rigidity secondary to TBI and reflecting on fluctuating hypertonicity*

Musculoskeletal Assessment

Musculoskeletal Assessment		Manual Muscle Test		Range of Motion	
		Right	Left	Right	Left
Shoulder	Flexors	NT	NT	WFL	WFL
	Extensors	NT	NT	WFL	WFL
	Abductors	NT	NT	15°	20°
	Adductors	NT	NT	0°	0°
	External Rotators	NT	NT	15°	15°
	Internal Rotators	NT	NT	-15°	-15°
Elbow	Flexors	NT	NT	WFL	WFL
	Extensors	NT	NT	-50°	-50°
Forearm	Pronators	NT	NT	75°	75°
	Supinators	NT	NT	-75°	-75°
Wrist	Flexors	NT	NT	NT	NT
	Extensors	NT	NT	-80°	-75°
Finger	Flexors/Hand Grip	NT	NT	-90°	-90°
Hip	Flexors	NT	NT	50°	56°
	Extensors	NT	NT	WFL	WFL
	Abductors	NT	NT	30°	33°
	Adductors	NT	NT	WFL	WFL
	External Rotators	NT	NT	-20°	-18°
	Internal Rotators	NT	NT	20°	20°

Musculoskeletal Assessment		Manual Muscle Test		Range of Motion	
		Right	Left	Right	Left
Knee	Flexors	NT	NT	38°	42°
	Extensors	NT	NT	WFL	WFL
Ankle	Dorsiflexors	NT	NT	-45°	-42°
	Plantar Flexors	NT	NT	45°	42°
Foot	Invertors	NT	NT	30°	30°
	Evertors	NT	NT	-30°	-30°

Musculoskeletal Assessment		ROM	MMT
Spine	Cervical Flexion	20°	NT
	Cervical Extension	-20°	NT
	Cervical Lateral Flexion (right)	-10°	NT
	Cervical Lateral Flexion (left)	15°	NT
	Cervical Rotation (right)	0°	NT
	Cervical Rotation (left)	0°	NT
	Lumbar Flexion	NT	NT
	Lumbar Extension	NT	NT
	Lumbar Lateral Flexion (right)	NT	NT
	Lumbar Lateral Flexion (left)	NT	NT

Evidence of Edema?   ☐ Yes   ■ No

Girth Anatomical Landmark: _____   ■ Not Applicable

Right:	_____inch(es)	Left:	_____ inch(es)

Leg-Length Discrepancy?   ☐ Yes   ■ No
Approximate Discrepancy: _____ inch(es)

Musculoskeletal Assessment (continued)

Posture	
Posture	❏ Normal Alignment ■ Postural Deviations Explain *Forward head, rt. cervical torticollis, internally rotated bilateral hips, kyphosis, bilateral equinovarus*

Spasmodic Activity					
	❏ No evidence of muscle spasms	**Grade**			
	■ Not applicable	1	2	3	4
Spasmodic Activity	**Muscles**				

Cardiopulmonary Assessment

Cardiopulmonary Assessment	
Lungs	❏ Clear to Auscultation ❏ Abnormal Breath Sounds ■ Adventitious Breath Sounds *Coarse rales at BLL* ❏ Resonant Chest to Mediate Percussion ❏ Other: ■ Bibasilar Thoracic Asymmetry *Decreased bibasilar; increased biapical* RR: _____ ❏ Normal ❏ Dyspnea ■ Other: *dc'd tracheostomy; closed (plugged) stoma*
Cardiac	■ Normal S1 Other: ■ Normal S2 ■ Split S1 ❏ Split S2 ❏ S3 ❏ S4 ❏ Murmur ❏ Ejection Click HR: _____ BP: _____

Neurological Assessment

Neurologic Assessment	
Superficial Sensation	❏ Intact **Explain** ❏ Impaired *Unable to test*
Coordination	❏ Intact **Explain** ❏ Impaired ❏ Intention Tremors *Unable to test*
Proprioception	❏ Intact **Explain** ❏ Impaired *Unable to test*
Deep Tendon Reflexes	❏ Intact **Explain** ❏ Diminished _____ ■ Hyperactive *patellar bilaterally* _____
Balance	Static ❏ Intact ❏ Impaired Dynamic ❏ Intact ❏ Impaired *Not tested*

Pain	No Pain Intolerable Pain 0 1 2 3 4 5 6 7 8 9 10 *c/o pain on passive range and stretch to knee flexors, hip flexors, ankle dorsiflexors bilaterally as well as horizontal abductors bilaterally but unable to estimate level.*
Tone	❏ Normal ■ Hypertonia / Spasticity *Severe BUE fluctuating flexor-extensor spasticity with prevalence of a flexor pattern; severe BLE extensor spasticity with occasional tone fluctuation in hip group* ❏ Hypotonia / Flaccidity ❏ Cogwheel Rigidity ■ Contractures *Early stages of contracture development in bilateral feet with evidence of equiovarus deformity; moderate onset of contractures noted in both hands*

Other Neurologic Test Results	**Check the Appropriate Box**			
		Pos	Neg	N/A
	SLR Test	❏	❏	■
	Neural Tension	❏	❏	■
	Ulnar Radial Median			
	Fabere Sign	❏	❏	■
	Compression Test	❏	❏	■
	Distraction Stretch	❏	❏	■
	Vertebral Artery Test	❏	❏	■
	Alar Ligament Test	❏	❏	■
	Vertebral Glide Test	❏	❏	■
	Babinski Sign	■	❏	❏
	Romberg's Test	❏	❏	■
	Other	❏	❏	■

Functional Assessment

Mobility	
Gait Analysis	❏ Ambulatory ■ Non-Ambulatory Explain: *pt. is wheelchair bound but requires assistance with wheelchair locomotion* ❏ Assistive Device: Weight Bearing: ❏ FWB ❏ PWB ❏ NWB ❏ No significant gait deviations noted. ■ Gait Deviations: *unable to evaluate* ■ Abnormal Gait
Bed Mobility	❏ Independent ■ Requires assistance ■ max ❏ mod ❏ min
Transfers	❏ Independent ■ Requires assistance ■ max ❏ mod ❏ min
Body Mechanics	■ Not tested ❏ Uses proper body mechanics when lifting, carrying, sitting, and lying down ❏ Does not use proper body mechanics when lifting, carrying, and lying down ❏ Needs further instruction and practice

Goals

❏ Improve endurance
❏ Improve balance
❏ Improve spinal mobility
■ Promote relaxation
■ Improve breathing patterns
Diaphragmatic and costolateral
❏ Decrease pain

❏ Increase muscle strength

❏ Increase joint range and flexibility

❏ Improve gait pattern
❏ Improve coordination and proprioception
❏ Reduce muscle fatigue
❏ Decrease edema and inflammation

❏ Improve postural alignment
❏ Improve circulation
❏ Improve motor control
■ Inhibit spasticity/hypertonicity
Extensor tone in BLE's and flexor tone in BUE's
❏ Resolution of muscle spasms:

Plan of Care

Frequency: _3_ times per week for _4_ weeks

Bad Ragaz	■ Passive Relaxation ❏ Passive Pelvic Tilts ❏ Pre-Gait ❏ Isotonic #1 ❏ Isotonic #2 ❏ Isometric ❏ Pre-Weight-Bearing ■ Tone Inhibition ❏ Passive Trunk Elongation/Knee Hold ❏ Passive Trunk Elongation/Pelvic Hold ■ Passive Trunk Elongation/Thoracic Hold ❏ Unilateral Upper Extremity ❏ Bilateral Upper Extremity ❏ Prone Unilateral Upper Extremity ❏ Unilateral Lower Extremity ❏ Bilateral Lower Extremity ■ Bilateral Symmetrical Lower Extremity #1 ❏ Bilateral Symmetrical Lower Extremity #2 ❏ Bilateral Reciprocal Lower Extremity ❏ Other: _____
Halliwick	❏ Phase I Adjustment ❏ Phase II Rotational Activities ❏ Turbulent Gliding ❏ Balance Training/Kangaroo Jumps ❏ Balance Training/Weight Shifting ■ Other: *Integrate modified and adapted ATNR in supine*

Cardiaquatics	❏ Level I Sequences: _____ Activities: ____
	❏ Level II Sequences: _____ Activities: ____
	❏ Level III Sequences: _____ Activities: ____
	❏ Level IV
	   ❏ Phase 1 ❏ Phase 2 ❏ Phase 3 ❏ All
	   ❏ Selected Sequences:

Other	❏ Applied Myofascial Release ❏ Deep Friction Massage ❏ Applied Joint Mobilization/Distraction ❏ Applied Spinal Mobilization/Distraction ❏ Applied Joint Approximation ❏ Applied Feldenkrais ❏ Applied Lymphatic Drainage ■ Watsu/Basic Flow ■ Watsu/Transitional Flow ❏ Clinical Wassertanzen I ❏ Clinical Wassertanzen II ❏ Clinical Wassertanzen III ❏ Applied Aquatic Craniosacral Therapy ❏ Trigger Point Therapy ❏ Ai Chi: _____ ❏ Spinal/Trunk Stabilization Protocol: ❏ Thoracic Outlet Syndrome Protocol: ■ Other: *Deep breathing and coughing techniques as needed before aquatic therapy session w/suctioning*

Functional / Goal Specific Aquatic Therapy Activities and Exercises

❏ Gait Training (Forward/Backward) Laps: _____
❏ Stair Climbing x _____
❏ Bicycling Reps: _____
❏ Prone Activities Min _____
❏ Aquajogging Laps: _____
❏ Heel Cord Stretch
❏ Iliopsoas Stretch
❏ Piriformis Stretch
❏ TFL Stretch
❏ IT Band Stretch
❏ Hip Add Stretch
❏ Stork Stand
❏ Front to Back Weight Shifting
❏ Side to Side Weight Shifting
❏ Heel Raises Reps: _____
❏ Four-Corner Pivot Reps: _____

❏ Side-Stepping Laps: _____
❏ Cross Over Stepping Laps: _____
❏ Deep-Water Stride Jump Reps: _____
❏ Deep-Water Jogging (fwd/retro): _____ min.
❏ Deep-Water Groin Stretch
❏ Knee to Chest Reps: _____
❏ Closed Kinematic Chain Exercises
❏ Deep-Water Double Knee Lifts Reps: _____
❏ Wall Slide Reps: _____
❏ Pelvic Tilts Reps: _____
❏ Supine Kicks Reps:_____
❏ Deep-Water Spinal Traction in Vertical Suspension
  (_____ lbs. x _____ min.)
❏ Resistive Exercises:
■ Other: *work on postural alignment in deep water using floatation devices*

Aquatic Work Conditioning

❏ Resistive Forward/Retro Gait x _____ laps
❏ Deep-Water Jogging (fwd/retro) x _____ min.
❏ Tethered Jogging # _____ x _____ min.
❏ Swimming: _____ laps/min

❏ Other:_____

Equipment Used

■ Bodyfit® Collar
❏ Floatation Vest
❏ Tire Tube
■ Floatation Pelvic Belt
❏ Fins
❏ Snorkel Mask
❏ Snorkel Tube
❏ Ankle Floats
❏ Aqua-Dumbbells

❏ AquaJogger
❏ Graduated-Resistance Paddles
❏ Hydrotone Boots
❏ Hoola Hoop
❏ Resistance Cord
❏ Thera-Band®
❏ Aquakinetic Machines
❏ Boards
❏ Floatation Noodle

❏ Hydrotone Dumbbells
❏ Weights: _____
■ Bad Ragaz Floatation Rings
❏ Swim Bar
❏ Recumbent Bicycle
❏ Underwater Treadmill
❏ Halliwick Blow Balls
❏ Other:_____

Adjunct Therapy

❏ Not Applicable

❏ Whirlpool: _____ min. (spa)
❏ Patient Education
❏ Posture and Body Mechanics
❏ Home Exercise Program

■ Other: *Chest Therapy as needed; Occupational therapy consult for serial splinting*

Land Based Therapy Treatments

❏ Not Applicable

Frequency: _____ times per week
          for _____ weeks
❏ US: _____
❏ ES: _____
❏ HP's: _____
❏ Massage: _____

❏ Therapeutic Exercises (specify):
❏ Paraffin Bath:
■ Cryotherapy: *Ice massage to plantar flexors, hip extensors, knee extensors, pectoral muscles, wrist flexors*
❏ Joint Mobilization:
❏ Piriformis Release

Comments: *Special precautions when pt. presents with increased retentional intrapulmonary secretions; advise not to treat in pool when congested and emphasize clearing tracheobronchial secretions.*

_____
Signature & Credentials of Therapist   Date

Discussion

Goniometric measurements in this patient show severe limitation due to the significant degree of spasticity present in the upper and lower extremities. Joints are beginning to show a fixed position suggesting contracture development, particularly in the hands and feet bilaterally. Documented postural deviations might be consistent with hypertonic spine extensors.

The extensive involvement of this case and the significant residual neuromuscular, cognitive, and functional deficits indicate the need for a passive approach. The therapist should focus on the application of tone-inhibiting techniques and interventions. However, other clinical problems might be addressed, such as postural alignment, with applied floatation devices in deep water. Serial splinting or serial casting is advised in order to increase range, stretch tight structures, decrease spasticity, and prevent the further development of contractures.

Since the patient presented with occasional bouts of pulmonary congestion that might be due to upper respiratory infections, this should be taken into consideration. When the congestion occurs, emphasis should be placed on stabilizing the respiratory problem as opposed to aquatic therapy. Exposing the patient to temperature changes in the water and in the environment might worsen the upper respiratory condition. If land therapy interventions such as chest therapy are applied under these circumstances, perhaps other cryotherapy techniques used to inhibit tone might be effective until the patient is safe to resume aquatic therapy.

Watsu® is a very effective intervention in achieving partial release of tone and allowing passive mobility.

Therefore, the aquatic therapy sessions should begin and end with a Watsu® session.

Halliwick rotational activities might be considered with the integration of the ATNR (asymmetrical tonic neck reflex) to inhibit contralateral hypertonicity.

Cerebrovascular Accidents

Cerebrovascular accidents (CVA), or strokes as they are commonly referred to, are the result of a sudden interruption or disruption of the arterial circulation to or within the brain resulting in ischemia or necrosis of the affected area or areas. The event generally involves one of the arterial vessels that form the Circle of Willis, which supplies blood to the brain. Most commonly, the middle cerebral artery is involved, but other arterial branches can and do become affected as well. Etiologically, a stroke can be caused by:

1. a thromboembolic episode
2. an aneurysm
3. ischemia from atherosclerosis of one of the vessels in the Circle of Willis
4. hemorrhage from a ruptured artery.

Some systemic conditions such as hypertension and high cholesterol have been identified as potential predisposing factors that can lead to a stroke. These are risk factors associated with cerebrovascular disease.

The clinical picture presented by the patient who has had a stroke is that of contralateral hemiplegia or hemiparesis. The decussation of tracts in the extrapyramidal system is responsible for this clinical manifestation. For instance, if a patient suffers a stroke secondary to occlusion of the right middle cerebral artery, the result will be a left-sided hemiplegia. Since the left hemisphere regulates speech, if the CVA occurs on the left middle cerebral artery, a right-sided hemiplegia will be accompanied by aphasia (loss or defects in the ability to speak). Other clinical signs such as hemianopsia (loss of peripheral vision) are also common but generally depend on the extent of cortical involvement. Body image problems such as the hemineglect syndrome will occur and generally interfere with the patient's rehabilitation process. Therefore, activities that enhance the awareness of the hemiplegic side should be integrated into the patient's plan of care.

In the acute stages following a CVA, the patient will exhibit flaccidity or paresis. Later, upper motor neuron signs begin to surface and spasticity develops. At this point, the onset of the synergies is imminent. In the upper extremity, the prevalence of a flexor synergy pattern is observed while the extensor synergy predominantly characterizes the lower extremity pattern. Involuntary reflexes and actions such as sneezing or yawning can elicit an increase in the intensity or severity of flexor and extensor synergy patterns. Brunnstrom refers to this phenomenon as the principle of associated reactions.

Therapy is one of the most significant aspects of the patient's rehabilitation. The primary clinical objective of therapy during the synergy stages is the inhibition of spasticity and the prevention of contractures. Land-based interventions include neurodevelopmental therapy, gait training, and balance training. The occupational therapist

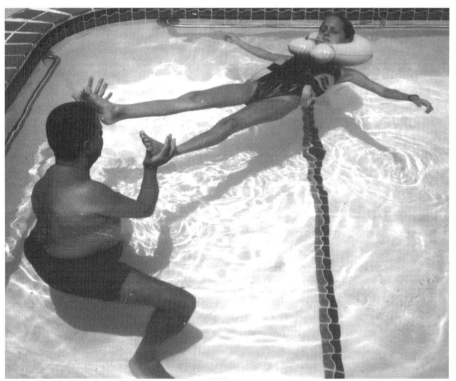

Figure 212: The applied Raimeste's technique.

works on the construction and application of splints that maintain range of motion and avoid an increase in hypertonicity.

When the patient is ready for aquatic rehabilitation, the therapist will complete a pre-aquatic assessment in order to establish goals and select the appropriate interventions. I recommend the application of the Raimeste's phenomenon principle in the water in an effort to facilitate motor activity in the involved side. This technique would elicit co-contraction of the hip abductors necessary for stability and gait. The applied Raimeste's technique consists of resisted abduction in the uninvolved side (Figure 212). However, the therapist's hands are placed at the lateral aspects of both ankles in order to palpate whether motor activity is elicited on the hemiplegic side. A flotation collar and pelvic belt will be needed for this technique.

Balance training is another clinical objective in aquatic rehabilitation. The integration of Halliwick Phase I balance and weight-shifting techniques is considered in the early stages of aquatic rehabilitation. Later, as improvement is noted in the patient's static and dynamic balance, more complex and challenging activities such the Halliwick Phase IV Kangaroo Jumps can be added.

The integration of selected Bad Ragaz Ring Method patterns could address upper and lower extremity motor deficits. The unilateral and bilateral upper extremity Bad Ragaz patterns are effective in the enhancement of neuromuscular reeducation, strength, and coordination in the upper limbs. If spasticity is a limiting factor, the Bad Ragaz passive relaxation position as well as the Bad Ragaz tone inhibition pattern would assist in decreasing tone.

Likewise, the Watsu® basic and transitional flow sequences are beneficially used as a tone-inhibiting approach. Additional techniques used effectively to reduce tone in the lower extremities include the Bad Ragaz trunk elongation patterns, particularly the pelvic hold technique. The rationale is that the hips are maintained in abduction with some degree of external rotation and slight knee flexion. This is an inhibiting position for lower extremity extensor spasticity. Furthermore, the Bad Ragaz bilateral symmetrical lower extremity #1 pattern would intensify these inhibiting motions thereby enhancing the reduction of tone.

Because of an increased relative density on the hemiplegic side, when placed in the supine position with floatation gear, the patient who has had a stroke has a tendency to roll toward the involved side. This manifestation is accentuated when the patient is asked to perform an activity such as a Bad Ragaz pattern and occurs secondary to a shift in the alignment of the metacenter in relation to the center of gravity. Halliwick Phase II rotational activities integrating chin and head control might help reduce the degree and extent of these unwanted rotations and facilitate motor control in the supine position.

CVA Case Study

The following case utilizes the DASI pre-aquatic assessment form to present clinical findings, establish goals, and select the interventions that would best meet the established goals. A discussion of the case is provided to justify the selection of activities, techniques, and interventions and to suggest other potentially effective strategies in the clinical management of the patient who has had a stroke.

DASI
Diagnostic Aquatics Systems Integration — Pre-Aquatic Therapy Assessment

Patient Name: ___*Bertha*_____   Date: _____

Dx: ___*Right- sided hemiparesis secondary to a left CVA of the middle cerebral artery*___   Age: __*58*_____

History/Problems/Complaints: *This patient is 2 years status post right CVA with residual. Pt received therapy during her acute and subacute phases of recovery both as an inpatient and as an outpatient.*

Clinical Impression: *Residual hemiplegia with balance impairment, weakness and gait deficits*

Musculoskeletal Assessment

Musculoskeletal Assessment		Manual Muscle Test		Range of Motion	
		Right	Left	Right	Left
Shoulder	Flexors	3-/5	5/5	WFL	WFL
	Extensors	3/5	5/5	WFL	WFL
	Abductors	3-/5	5/5	WFL	WFL
	Adductors	3/5	5/5	WFL	WFL
	External Rotators	3-/5	5/5	WFL	WFL
	Internal Rotators	3/5	5/5	WFL	WFL
Elbow	Flexors	3-/5	5/5	WFL	WFL
	Extensors	3/5	5/5	WFL	WFL
Forearm	Pronators	3+/5	5/5	WFL	WFL
	Supinators	3/5	5/5	WFL	WFL
Wrist	Flexors	3+/5	5/5	WFL	WFL
	Extensors	2/5	5/5	WFL	WFL
Finger	Flexors/Hand Grip	2/5	5/5	WFL	WFL
Hip	Flexors	2/5	4/5	WFL	WFL
	Extensors	3-/5	4/5	WFL	WFL
	Abductors	2+/5	4/5	WFL	WFL
	Adductors	3/5	4/5	WFL	WFL
	External Rotators	3-/5	4/5	WFL	WFL
	Internal Rotators	3-/5	4/5	WFL	WFL

Musculoskeletal Assessment		Manual Muscle Test		Range of Motion	
		Right	Left	Right	Left
Knee	Flexors	3/5	4/5	WFL	WFL
	Extensors	3+/5	4/5	WFL	WFL
Ankle	Dorsiflexors	2/5	4/5	-30°	WFL
	Plantar Flexors	3+/5	4/5	WFL	WFL
Foot	Invertors	3/5	4/5	WFL	WFL
	Evertors	3-/5	4/5	10°	WFL

Musculoskeletal Assessment	ROM	MMT
Cervical Flexion	35°	4+/5
Cervical Extension	-20°	4/5
Cervical Lateral Flexion (right)	5°	4/5
Cervical Lateral Flexion (left)	5°	4/5
Cervical Rotation (right)	5°	4/5
Cervical Rotation (left)	5°	4/5
Lumbar Flexion	Not tested	4-/5
Lumbar Extension	Not tested	4-/5
Lumbar Lateral Flexion (right)	Not tested	4-/5
Lumbar Lateral Flexion (left)	Not tested	4-/5

(Spine)

Evidence of Edema?　☐ Yes　■ No

Leg-Length Discrepancy?　■ Yes　☐ No
Approximate Discrepancy: _*1.5*_____ inch(es)

Girth Anatomical Landmark: _____ ■ Not Applicable		
Right:	_____inch(es)	Left:	_____ inch(es)

Cardiopulmonary Assessment

Musculoskeletal Assessment (continued)

Posture

Posture

- ☐ Normal Alignment
- ■ Postural Deviations

Explain *Forward head, round shoulders, kyphoscoliosis, moderate equinovarus*

Spasmodic Activity

☐ No evidence of muscle spasms	Grade			
■ Not applicable	1	2	3	4

Spasmodic Activity

Muscles				

Cardiopulmonary Assessment

Lungs

- ■ Clear to Auscultation
- ☐ Abnormal Breath Sounds
- ☐ Adventitious Breath Sounds
- ■ Resonant Chest to Mediate Percussion
- ☐ Other:
- ☐ Bibasilar Thoracic Asymmetry

RR: _____ ■ Normal ☐ Dyspnea ☐ Other:

Cardiac

	Other:
■ Normal S1 ■ Normal S2 ☐ Split S1 ☐ Split S2 ☐ S3 ☐ S4 ☐ Murmur ☐ Ejection Click HR: 72 BP: 138/88	

Neurological Assessment

Neurologic Assessment

Superficial Sensation

- ☐ Intact   **Explain**
- ■ Impaired

rt. shoulder, dorsum of rt. forearm, RLE

Coordination

- ☐ Intact   **Explain**
- ■ Impaired
- ☐ Intention Tremors

Deficits noted in bilateral upper and lower extremities

Proprioception

- ☐ Intact   **Explain**
- ■ Impaired

Impaired kinesthesia in both upper and lower extremities

Deep Tendon Reflexes

- ☐ Intact   **Explain**
- ■ Diminished *rt. biceps and patellar*
- ☐ Hyperactive _____

Balance

Static	☐ Intact	■ Impaired
Dynamic	☐ Intact	■ Impaired

Pain

No Pain   Intolerable Pain

0 1■ 2   3   4   5   6   7   8   9   10

rt. shoulder

Tone

- ☐ Normal
- ■ Hypertonia / Spasticity

Extensor tone in LE's; flexor tone in UE's

- ☐ Hypotonia / Flaccidity
- ☐ Cogwheel Rigidity
- ☐ Contractures

Other Neurologic Test Results

	Check the Appropriate Box		
	Pos	Neg	N/A
SLR Test	☐	☐	■
Neural Tension	☐	☐	■
	Ulnar	Radial	Median
Fabere Sign	☐	☐	■
Compression Test	☐	☐	■
Distraction Stretch	☐	☐	■
Vertebral Artery Test	■	☐	☐
Alar Ligament Test	☐	☐	■
Vertebral Glide Test	☐	☐	■
Babinski Sign	☐	☐	■
Romberg's Test	■	☐	☐
Other *Positive clonus on rt. foot/ankle*	■	☐	☐

Functional Assessment

Mobility		
Gait Analysis	■ Ambulatory ❏ Non-Ambulatory Explain: *Wears rt. arm sling* ■ Assistive Device: *Quad Cane* Weight Bearing: ■ FWB ❏ PWB ❏ NWB ❏ No significant gait deviations noted. ■ Gait Deviations: *Evidence of a moderate Trendelenburg's gait with moderate steppage gait* ■ Abnormal Gait *Hikes rt. hip on swing phase with inward rotation on heel strike and knee flexion in preparation for stance*	
Bed Mobility	❏ Independent ■ Requires assistance ❏ max ❏ mod ■ min	
Transfers	■ Independent ❏ Requires assistance ❏ max ❏ mod ❏ min	
Body Mechanics	■ Not tested ❏ Uses proper body mechanics when lifting, carrying, sitting, and lying down ❏ Does not use proper body mechanics when lifting, carrying, and lying down ❏ Needs further instruction and practice	

Goals
■ Improve endurance
■ Improve balance
❏ Improve spinal mobility
■ Promote relaxation
❏ Improve breathing patterns

___

■ Decrease pain
rt. shoulder
■ Increase muscle strength
on muscle groups with documented weakness
■ Increase joint range and flexibility *on joints and movements with documented limitations*
■ Improve gait pattern
■ Improve coordination and proprioception
❏ Reduce muscle fatigue
❏ Decrease edema and inflammation

___

■ Improve postural alignment
❏ Improve circulation
■ Improve motor control
■ Inhibit spasticity/hypertonicity
Extensor tone in BLE's and flexor tone in BUE's
❏ Resolution of muscle spasms:

___

Plan of Care

Frequency: _3_ times per week for _4_ weeks

Bad Ragaz	
Bad Ragaz	■ Passive Relaxation ❏ Passive Pelvic Tilts ❏ Pre-Gait ❏ Isotonic #1 ❏ Isotonic #2 ❏ Isometric ❏ Pre-Weight-Bearing ■ Tone Inhibition ■ Passive Trunk Elongation/Knee Hold ■ Passive Trunk Elongation/Pelvic Hold ■ Passive Trunk Elongation/Thoracic Hold ■ Unilateral Upper Extremity ■ Bilateral Upper Extremity ❏ Prone Unilateral Upper Extremity ❏ Unilateral Lower Extremity ❏ Bilateral Lower Extremity ■ Bilateral Symmetrical Lower Extremity #1 ❏ Bilateral Symmetrical Lower Extremity #2 ❏ Bilateral Reciprocal Lower Extremity ■ Other: *Applied Raimeste's Technique for rt. hip abductors*
Halliwick	❏ Phase I Adjustment ■ Phase II Rotational Activities ❏ Turbulent Gliding ■ Balance Training/Kangaroo Jumps ■ Balance Training/Weight Shifting ❏ Other: _____

Cardiaquatics	❏ Level I Sequences: ___ Activities: ___
	❏ Level II Sequences: ___ Activities: ___
	❏ Level III Sequences: ___ Activities: ___
	❏ Level IV
	   ❏ Phase 1 ❏ Phase 2 ❏ Phase 3 ❏ All
	   ❏ Selected Sequences:

Other	❏ Applied Myofascial Release ❏ Deep Friction Massage ❏ Applied Joint Mobilization/Distraction ❏ Applied Spinal Mobilization/Distraction ❏ Applied Joint Approximation ❏ Applied Feldenkrais ❏ Applied Lymphatic Drainage ■ Watsu/Basic Flow ■ Watsu/Transitional Flow ❏ Clinical Wassertanzen I ❏ Clinical Wassertanzen II ❏ Clinical Wassertanzen III ❏ Applied Aquatic Craniosacral Therapy ❏ Trigger Point Therapy ❏ Ai Chi: _____ ❏ Spinal/Trunk Stabilization Protocol: ❏ Thoracic Outlet Syndrome Protocol: ❏ Other: _____

Functional / Goal Specific Aquatic Therapy Activities and Exercises

■ Gait Training (<u>Forward</u>/Backward) Laps: *3*
■ Stair Climbing x *2*___
❏ Bicycling Reps: ____
❏ Prone Activities Min ____
❏ Aquajogging Laps: ____
❏ Heel Cord Stretch
❏ Iliopsoas Stretch
❏ Piriformis Stretch
❏ TFL Stretch
❏ IT Band Stretch
❏ Hip Add Stretch
■ Stork Stand
❏ Front to Back Weight Shifting
❏ Side to Side Weight Shifting
❏ Heel Raises Reps: ____
■ Four-Corner Pivot Reps: *2*___

■ Side-Stepping Laps: *3*___
❏ Cross Over Stepping Laps: ____
❏ Deep-Water Stride Jump Reps: ____
❏ Deep-Water Jogging (fwd/retro): ____ min.
❏ Deep-Water Groin Stretch
❏ Knee to Chest Reps: ____
❏ Closed Kinematic Chain Exercises
❏ Deep-Water Double Knee Lifts Reps: ____
❏ Wall Slide Reps: ____
❏ Pelvic Tilts Reps: ___
❏ Supine Kicks Reps:____
❏ Deep-Water Spinal Traction in Vertical Suspension
  (____ lbs. x ____ min.)
❏ Resistive Exercises:

■ Other: *Side-Stepping Crab Walk x 3 laps* ____

Aquatic Work Conditioning

❏ Resistive Forward/Retro Gait x ____ laps
❏ Deep-Water Jogging (fwd/retro) x ____ min.
❏ Tethered Jogging # ____ x ____ min.
❏ Swimming: ____ laps/min

❏ Other:_____

Equipment Used

■ Bodyfit® Collar
❏ Floatation Vest
❏ Tire Tube
■ Floatation Pelvic Belt
❏ Fins
❏ Snorkel Mask
❏ Snorkel Tube
❏ Ankle Floats
❏ Aqua-Dumbbells

❏ AquaJogger
❏ Graduated-Resistance Paddles
❏ Hydrotone Boots
❏ Hoola Hoop
❏ Resistance Cord
❏ Thera-Band®
❏ Aquakinetic Machines
❏ Boards
❏ Floatation Noodle

❏ Hydrotone Dumbbells
❏ Weights: ____
■ Bad Ragaz Floatation Rings
❏ Swim Bar
❏ Recumbent Bicycle
❏ Underwater Treadmill
❏ Halliwick Blow Balls
❏ Other:_____

Adjunct Therapy

■ Not Applicable

❏ Whirlpool: ____ min. (spa)
❏ Patient Education
❏ Posture and Body Mechanics
❏ Home Exercise Program

❏ Other:_____

Land Based Therapy Treatments

❏ Not Applicable

Frequency: ____ times per week
        for ____ weeks
❏ US: _____
❏ ES: _____
❏ HP's: _____
❏ Massage: _____

❏ Therapeutic Exercises (specify):
❏ Paraffin Bath:
■ Cryotherapy: *Ice massage to rt.*
elbow and wrist flexor, hip and knee
extensors, ankle plantar flexors, as
needed
❏ Joint Mobilization:
❏ Piriformis Release

Comments:

_____   _____

Signature & Credentials of Therapist   Date

Discussion

Despite prior rehabilitation, Bertha still demonstrates significant weakness of the involved side. Although there is no evidence of contractures, she shows limitations in range of motion due to residual spasticity and tightness of the connective tissue. Aquatic therapy will focus on neuromuscular reeducation of the hemiparetic side while at the same time integrating tone inhibition techniques. Besides reducing tone and promoting relaxation, Watsu® could potentially be beneficial in improving superficial sensation through tactile stimulus. The same is true of selected Bad Ragaz patterns. The application of Bad Ragaz patterns will further address other clinical problems such as coordination, kinesthesia, and weak muscle groups. Selected patterns should first be applied passively and without resistance. Resistance can be added once improvement is noticed or upon the discretion of the therapist.

Working on static and dynamic balance is a fundamental consideration for gait training. Balance training techniques should begin with basic activities, progressing to more complex and challenging ones once motor control and balance improve. Static balance activities such as the stork stand set the tone for dynamic balance activities, which would precede gait training. The side-stepping crab walk with a short or long arm hold addresses dynamic balance problems and gait deficits.

Application of chin and head control techniques in Halliwick sagittal rotations with the patient in the vertical upright position might help in reducing the effects of increased relative density of the hemiparetic side. Phase II rotations should also be practiced in the supine position.

Spinal Cord Injury

The clinical picture and manifestations associated with the patient who has sustained a spinal cord injury vary according to the severity and type of injury, e.g., complete transection versus incomplete injury. A patient with complete transection of the spinal cord presents a flaccid paralysis with total loss of motor and sensory function below the level of injury. If the injury involves the cervical spine, this reflects in quadriplegia or paralysis of the four extremities and the trunk musculature. If the spine is transected at T12, the clinical picture is that of a paraplegia or paralysis of the lower extremities. The higher the level of injury, the more significant and extensive the motor, sensory, and systemic problems encountered. Paralysis of the respiratory muscles requiring mechanical ventilation occurs in the patient with high quadriplegia. Immediately following the spinal shock and acute stages of the injury, there is flaccid paralysis with areflexia. Once the localized edema and inflammation have subsided around the site of cord transection, a gradual increase in muscle tone begins to develop along with hyperreflexia. This upper motor neuron sign is referred to as spasticity or hypertonicity. The most commonly seen patterns of spasticity consist of lower extremity extensor spasticity and upper extremity flexor spasticity. However, at the level of the injury, lower motor neuron signs such as motor paresis and atrophy are also manifested. Autonomic pathways are also involved reflecting in bowel and bladder dysfunction.

Incomplete lesions will present a different clinical picture. These generally consist of an anterior, posterior, or lateral hemisection of the spinal cord. If the cord sustains a lateral hemisection, there will be ipsilateral loss of proprioception and motor function with contralateral loss of pain and temperature. This is referred to as Brown-Séquard syndrome. Because of the decussation of the spinothalamic and corticospinal tracts, patients with incomplete lesions will also exhibit other sensorimotor deficits such as vibratory sense, pain, temperature, proprioception, and motor control.

Etiologically speaking, spinal cord injuries are most frequently caused by trauma. However, secondary causes include neoplasms, spinal hematomas or abscesses, parainfectious syndromes, herniated intervertebral discs, and multiple sclerosis.

Aquatic rehabilitation offers some benefits for the patient who has sustained a spinal cord injury (SCI). However, the therapist must exercise caution given the type of SCI and considering a complete versus incomplete lesion. If the patient has been physiologically unstable, it is best to wait until full clearance from the physician is received. Physiologic instability could reflect in frequent bouts of autonomic dysreflexia. The presence of autonomic dysreflexia generally suggests cardiovascular, gastrointestinal, or renal problems but it may also result from other causes such as inappropriate position of an extremity or occlusion of the Foley catheter. The manifestations of autonomic dysreflexia include high blood pressure above the injury (which may lead to stroke), diaphoresis above the level of the spinal injury, lightheadedness or dizziness, nausea, and a sudden drop in blood pressure below the level of the spinal cord injury. Prior to the aquatic therapy session, all bowel and bladder procedures should have been performed. Patients with paraplegia generally do not experience this type of problem.

A patient with a spinal cord injury who has an indwelling catheter in place should not be treated in the pool. Another contraindication for pool therapy is evidence of decubiti. Skin inspection by the therapist on a daily basis is extremely important. Floatation equipment should be applied prior to transferring the patient into the pool. Patients with paraplegia can be transferred into the pool via a hydraulic chair or mechanical lift chair. Patients with quadriplegia require a mechanical lift with a stretcher for transfer into the pool. Some pools are equipped with ramps that allow a patient with quadriplegia to be transported into the pool in a wheelchair. Should this be the case, the wheelchairs used must be specially designed and manufactured for transportation into the pool.

The most significant clinical goal in aquatic therapy for a patient who has sustained a spinal cord injury is to decrease tone. The application of Watsu® basic and transitional flow sequences can prove effective in reducing hypertonicity, maintaining joint flexibility, and promoting relaxation. For the patient with paraplegia, additional functional goals could include the attainment of upright balance and maintenance or increase of muscle strength in the upper extremities and trunk. Selected Bad Ragaz Ring Method patterns such as the bilateral upper extremity can be applied for this purpose. When trunk control, postural alignment, and balance are emphasized, deep-water activities may be added. Halliwick Phase II chin and head control techniques can be effective in improving posture and attaining balance in the upright position. Paraplegics exhibit an increased relative density in the lower extremities. Therefore, when supine activities are considered, ankle floats should be used in addition to other floatation devices. Upright standing activities in shallow water might require additional support. The Halliwick short- or long-arm hold might prove helpful while still allowing the patient to recruit the necessary trunk musculature for functional standing and balance activities.

Spinal Cord Injury Case Study

The following case utilizes the DASI pre-aquatic assessment form to present clinical findings, establish goals, and select the interventions that would best meet the established goals. A discussion of the case is provided to justify the selection of activities, techniques, and interventions and to suggest other potentially effective strategies in the clinical management of the SCI patient.

DASI
Diagnostic Aquatics Systems Integration — Pre-Aquatic Therapy Assessment

Patient Name: _____*Mickey*_____   Date: _____

Dx: ___*L4-L5 Paraplegia secondary to motorcycle accident*_____   Age: ___*24*_____

History/Problems/Complaints: *This young man sustained a motorcycle accident a year and a half ago resulting in a complete transection of the spinal cord at L4-L5. Mickey was and remains very active in sports and athletic activities. He was an avid swimmer before his accident and currently participates in wheelchair marathons. He underwent a rigorous course of rehabilitation following his injury. Currently, he is on intermittent catheterization, which he performs on a regularly established scheduled.*
Clinical Impression: *Residual L4-L5 paraplegia*

Musculoskeletal Assessment

Musculoskeletal Assessment		Manual Muscle Test		Range of Motion	
		Right	Left	Right	Left
Shoulder	Flexors	5/5	5/5	WFL	WFL
	Extensors	5/5	5/5	WFL	WFL
	Abductors	5/5	5/5	WFL	WFL
	Adductors	5/5	5/5	WFL	WFL
	External Rotators	5/5	5/5	WFL	WFL
	Internal Rotators	5/5	5/5	WFL	WFL
Elbow	Flexors	5/5	5/5	WFL	WFL
	Extensors	5/5	5/5	WFL	WFL
Forearm	Pronators	5/5	5/5	WFL	WFL
	Supinators	5/5	5/5	WFL	WFL
Wrist	Flexors	5/5	5/5	WFL	WFL
	Extensors	5/5	5/5	WFL	WFL
Finger	Flexors/Hand Grip	5/5	5/5	WFL	WFL
Hip	Flexors	3/5	3/5	WFL	WFL
	Extensors	0/5	0/5	WFL	WFL
	Abductors	2+/5	2+/5	WFL	WFL
	Adductors	3/5	3/5	WFL	WFL
	External Rotators	2/5	2/5	WFL	WFL
	Internal Rotators	3/5	3/5	WFL	WFL

Musculoskeletal Assessment		Manual Muscle Test		Range of Motion	
		Right	Left	Right	Left
Knee	Flexors	2-/5	2-/5	WFL	WFL
	Extensors	3-/5	3-/5	WFL	WFL
Ankle	Dorsiflexors	2-/5	2-/5	WFL	WFL
	Plantar Flexors	2-/5	2-/5	WFL	WFL
Foot	Invertors	2/5	2/5	WFL	WFL
	Evertors	2-/5	2/5	WFL	WFL

Musculoskeletal Assessment	ROM	MMT
Cervical Flexion	WFL	5/5
Cervical Extension	WFL	5/5
Cervical Lateral Flexion (right)	WFL	5/5
Cervical Lateral Flexion (left)	WFL	5/5
Cervical Rotation (right)	WFL	5/5
Cervical Rotation (left)	WFL	5/5
Lumbar Flexion	WFL	5/5
Lumbar Extension	WFL	5/5
Lumbar Lateral Flexion (right)	WFL	5/5
Lumbar Lateral Flexion (left)	WFL	5/5

(Spine)

Evidence of Edema?   ❑ Yes   ■ No

Girth Anatomical Landmark: ____ ■ Not Applicable

Right:	_____inch(es)	Left:	_____ inch(es)

Leg-Length Discrepancy?   ❑ Yes   ■ No
Approximate Discrepancy: _____ inch(es)

Musculoskeletal Assessment (continued)

Posture

Posture	❏ Normal Alignment ■ Postural Deviations Explain *Lumbar lordosis, Genu Recurvatum*

Spasmodic Activity

❏ No evidence of muscle spasms ■ Not applicable		**Grade**			
		1	2	3	4

	Muscles				
Spasmodic Activity					

Cardiopulmonary Assessment

Cardiopulmonary Assessment

Lungs	■ Clear to Auscultation ❏ Abnormal Breath Sounds ❏ Adventitious Breath Sounds ■ Resonant Chest to Mediate Percussion ❏ Other: ❏ Bibasilar Thoracic Asymmetry RR: _____ ■ Normal ❏ Dyspnea ❏ Other:
Cardiac	■ Normal S1 Other: ■ Normal S2 ❏ Split S1 ❏ Split S2 ❏ S3 ❏ S4 ❏ Murmur ❏ Ejection Click HR: _72_ BP: _138/88_

Neurological Assessment

Neurologic Assessment

Superficial Sensation	❏ Intact **Explain** ■ Impaired *Lateral aspects of both legs and ankle; dorsum of feet bilaterally*
Coordination	■ Intact **Explain** ❏ Impaired ❏ Intention Tremors *Intact but noticeably weak in the lower extremities*
Proprioception	❏ Intact **Explain** ■ Impaired *Impaired kinesthesia in both lower extremities*
Deep Tendon Reflexes	❏ Intact **Explain** ■ Diminished *bilateral patellar (almost areflexic)* ❏ Hyperactive _____
Balance	Static ■ Intact ❏ Impaired Dynamic ■ Intact ❏ Impaired

Pain	No Pain Intolerable Pain ■ 1 2 3 4 5 6 7 8 9 10
Tone	❏ Normal ■ Hypertonia / Spasticity *Fluctuating tone in BLE's; bilateral clonus* ❏ Hypotonia / Flaccidity ❏ Cogwheel Rigidity ❏ Contractures

	Check the Appropriate Box		
Other Neurologic Test Results		Pos	Neg	N/A
SLR Test	❏	❏	■
Neural Tension	❏	❏	■
	Ulnar Radial Median		
Fabere Sign	❏	❏	■
Compression Test	❏	❏	■
Distraction Stretch	❏	❏	■
Vertebral Artery Test	❏	❏	■
Alar Ligament Test	❏	❏	■
Vertebral Glide Test	❏	❏	■
Babinski Sign	■	❏	❏
Romberg's Test	❏	❏	■
Other	■	❏	❏
Positive clonus on bilateral ankles/feet			

Functional Assessment

	Mobility
Gait Analysis	■ Ambulatory ❑ Non-Ambulatory Explain: *pt. ambulates with Lofstrand crutches and long leg braces; occasionally wears KAFO; occasionally uses wheelchair as ambulatory means* ■ Assistive Device: *Lofstrand crutches, long leg braces: KAFO; standard wheelchair* Weight Bearing: ■ FWB ❑ PWB ❑ NWB ❑ No significant gait deviations noted. ■ Gait Deviations: *bilateral hip hiking on midswing* ■ Abnormal Gait *Hikes bilateral hip on swing phase with inward rotation; uses four point alternate gait pattern*
Bed Mobility	❑ Independent ■ Requires assistance ❑ max ❑ mod ■ min
Transfers	■ Independent ❑ Requires assistance ❑ max ❑ mod ❑ min
Body Mechanics	■ Not tested ❑ Uses proper body mechanics when lifting, carrying, sitting, and lying down ❑ Does not use proper body mechanics when lifting, carrying, and lying down ❑ Needs further instruction and practice

Goals

■ Improve endurance
❑ Improve balance
❑ Improve spinal mobility
■ Promote relaxation
❑ Improve breathing patterns

❑ Decrease pain

■ Increase muscle strength
on muscle groups with documented weakness
❑ Increase joint range and flexibility

■ Improve gait pattern
■ Improve coordination and proprioception
❑ Reduce muscle fatigue
❑ Decrease edema and inflammation

❑ Improve postural alignment
❑ Improve circulation
■ Improve motor control
■ Inhibit spasticity/hypertonicity
fluctuating tone in BLE's as documented
❑ Resolution of muscle spasms:

Plan of Care

Frequency: __3__ times per week for __4__ weeks

Bad Ragaz	■ Passive Relaxation ❑ Passive Pelvic Tilts ❑ Pre-Gait ❑ Isotonic #1 ❑ Isotonic #2 ❑ Isometric ❑ Pre-Weight-Bearing ■ Tone Inhibition ■ Passive Trunk Elongation/Knee Hold ■ Passive Trunk Elongation/Pelvic Hold ■ Passive Trunk Elongation/Thoracic Hold ■ Unilateral Upper Extremity ■ Bilateral Upper Extremity ❑ Prone Unilateral Upper Extremity ❑ Unilateral Lower Extremity ■ Bilateral Lower Extremity ■ Bilateral Symmetrical Lower Extremity #1 ❑ Bilateral Symmetrical Lower Extremity #2 ❑ Bilateral Reciprocal Lower Extremity ❑ Other: _____
Halliwick	❑ Phase I Adjustment ■ Phase II Rotational Activities ❑ Turbulent Gliding ❑ Balance Training/Kangaroo Jumps ■ Balance Training/Weight Shifting ❑ Other: _____

Cardiaquatics	❑ Level I Sequences: _____ Activities: ____
	❑ Level II Sequences: _____ Activities: ____
	❑ Level III Sequences: _____ Activities: ____
	❑ Level IV
	    ❑ Phase 1 ❑ Phase 2 ❑ Phase 3 ❑ All
	    ❑ Selected Sequences:

Other	❑ Applied Myofascial Release ❑ Deep Friction Massage ❑ Applied Joint Mobilization/Distraction ❑ Applied Spinal Mobilization/Distraction ❑ Applied Joint Approximation ❑ Applied Feldenkrais ❑ Applied Lymphatic Drainage ❑ Watsu/Basic Flow ■ Watsu/Transitional Flow ■ Clinical Wassertanzen I ■ Clinical Wassertanzen II ■ Clinical Wassertanzen III ❑ Applied Aquatic Craniosacral Therapy ❑ Trigger Point Therapy ❑ Ai Chi: _____ ❑ Spinal/Trunk Stabilization Protocol: _____ ❑ Thoracic Outlet Syndrome Protocol: _____ ❑ Other: _____

Functional / Goal Specific Aquatic Therapy Activities and Exercises

- [x] Gait Training (Forward/Backward) Laps: *3*____
- [ ] Stair Climbing x ____
- [ ] Bicycling Reps: ____
- [ ] Prone Activities Min ____
- [ ] Aquajogging Laps: ____
- [ ] Heel Cord Stretch
- [ ] Iliopsoas Stretch
- [ ] Piriformis Stretch
- [ ] TFL Stretch
- [ ] IT Band Stretch
- [ ] Hip Add Stretch
- [ ] Stork Stand
- [ ] Front to Back Weight Shifting
- [ ] Side to Side Weight Shifting
- [ ] Heel Raises Reps: ____
- [ ] Four-Corner Pivot Reps: ____

- [x] Side-Stepping Laps: *3*____
- [ ] Cross Over Stepping Laps: ____
- [ ] Deep-Water Stride Jump Reps: ____
- [ ] Deep-Water Jogging (fwd/retro): ____ min.
- [ ] Deep-Water Groin Stretch
- [ ] Knee to Chest Reps: ____
- [ ] Closed Kinematic Chain Exercises
- [ ] Deep-Water Double Knee Lifts Reps: ____
- [ ] Wall Slide Reps: ____
- [ ] Pelvic Tilts Reps: ___
- [ ] Supine Kicks Reps: ____
- [ ] Deep-Water Spinal Traction in Vertical Suspension (____ lbs. x ____ min.)
- [x] Resistive Exercises: *BUE's*

- [x] Other: *Side-Stepping Crab Walk x 3 laps*

Aquatic Work Conditioning

- [ ] Resistive Forward/Retro Gait x ____ laps
- [ ] Deep-Water Jogging (fwd/retro) x ____ min.
- [ ] Tethered Jogging # ____ x ____ min.
- [x] Swimming: *1-2*____ laps/min

- [ ] Other:____

Equipment Used

- [x] Bodyfit® Collar
- [ ] Floatation Vest
- [ ] Tire Tube
- [x] Floatation Pelvic Belt
- [ ] Fins
- [x] Snorkel Mask
- [ ] Snorkel Tube
- [x] Ankle Floats
- [ ] Aqua-Dumbbells

- [ ] AquaJogger
- [ ] Graduated-Resistance Paddles
- [ ] Hydrotone Boots
- [ ] Hoola Hoop
- [ ] Resistance Cord
- [ ] Thera-Band®
- [ ] Aquakinetic Machines
- [ ] Boards
- [x] Floatation Noodle

- [ ] Hydrotone Dumbbells
- [ ] Weights: ____
- [x] Bad Ragaz Floatation Rings
- [ ] Swim Bar
- [ ] Recumbent Bicycle
- [ ] Underwater Treadmill
- [x] Halliwick Blow Balls
- [x] Other: *Adapted BLE Braces for pool therapy use only*

Adjunct Therapy

- [x] Not Applicable
- [ ] Whirlpool: ____ min. (spa)

- [ ] Patient Education
- [ ] Posture and Body Mechanics

- [ ] Home Exercise Program
- [ ] Other:____

Land Based Therapy Treatments

- [ ] Not Applicable

Frequency: ____ times per week for ____ weeks
- [ ] US: ____
- [ ] ES: ____

- [ ] HP's: ____
- [ ] Massage: ____
- [ ] Piriformis Release
- [ ] Therapeutic Exercises (specify):
- [ ] Paraffin Bath:

- [x] Cryotherapy: *Ice massage to hip and knee extensors, ankle plantar flexors as needed*
- [ ] Joint Mobilization:
- [ ] Other:

Comments:

____

Signature & Credentials of Therapist   Date

Discussion

In this case, Mickey remains very active and physically fit considering his paraplegia. He has optimal strength in his upper extremities, shoulder girdle, scapular muscles, and abdominal muscles, which will allow him to integrate swimming laps into his aquatic rehabilitation program. Resistive exercises using weights or aqua dumbbells with the patient sitting on a bench is an effective treatment technique for upper extremity strengthening. Prone swimming activities or selected interventions performed in the supine position might require the use of ankle floats because lower extremity paralysis with episodes of fluctuating tone will increase the relative density causing the lower limbs to sink.

Bad Ragaz upper extremity patterns should integrate resistance to maintain strength and coordination. Bad Ragaz lower extremity patterns should focus on inhibition of spasticity, range of motion, and flexibility. When tone is unusually high, the therapist might consider cryotherapy methods using ice massage prior to the aquatic therapy session. Maintaining strength in the abdominal and back muscles can be achieved through the application of selected Bad Ragaz passive trunk elongation patterns, which integrate alternate stretch reflex facilitation. These patterns along with the integration of Halliwick rotational activities in deep water enhance motor control in the trunk and upper quarter.

The application of interventions such as Watsu® and the Clinical Wassertanzen Protocol are indicated in this patient to maintain optimal tidal volume and vital capacity, to promote relaxation, and to decrease tone in the lower extremities. Considering that this patient was and remains very active in athletic activities, he should able to complete the three phases of the Clinical Wassertanzen Protocol.

Other dynamic shallow-water activities might help in the improvement of posture and gait. If possible, a set of long leg braces should be used exclusively for aquatic therapy purposes or a KAFO should be fabricated especially for gait activities in shallow water. Gait training may be practiced on parallel bars, if these are available, or by applying the Halliwick long-arm hold technique for support and contact guarding.

Multiple Sclerosis

Multiple sclerosis (MS) is a progressive neurological disorder characterized by patches of demyelination developing in the brain, brainstem, cerebellum, and spinal cord. Visual disturbances, sensory impairment, weakness of the extremities, and problems with coordination are common initial signs of this disease. Most patients experience ongoing periods of remission and exacerbation throughout the course of the disease. The pathogenesis of multiple sclerosis has been attributed to abnormalities in the individual's immunologic system. Even though there is still much debate about the etiology of multiple sclerosis, epidemiologic studies suggest that viral infections may be the primary cause. Secondary causes may include genetic and environmental factors.

Involvement of the pyramidal tracts, particularly the corticospinal tract, leads to the onset of upper motor neuron signs such as spasticity, hyperreflexia, and a positive Babinski sign. Cerebellar involvement results in nystagmus and ataxia. However, the most common complaint expressed by the patient with MS is muscle fatigue, which is described as severe exhaustion interfering with the patient's daily activities. The degree of severity of this illness can range from a mild form to a severe form. In the mild form the patient remains ambulatory with or without assistive devices throughout the course of the disease. In the severe form, the patient might be wheelchair bound exhibiting possible deformities and contractures as a result of severe hypertonia.

Environmental factors have a tendency to contribute to the exacerbation or remission of multiple sclerosis. An increase in temperature tends to elicit, influence, or intensify the clinical manifestations that characterize this disease. In the 1970s a diagnostic procedure called the Hot Bath Test Procedure was used for patients who were suspected to be in the early stages of MS. This test was performed in the physical therapy department using the Hubbard tank. The neurologist, a nurse, and the physical therapist were present. The patient was placed in the Hubbard tank via the mechanical lift. The temperature of the water was maintained at 102°F. The water surface level was covered with a transparent vinyl sheet to contain the heat, leaving only the patient's head and neck uncovered. The oral temperature of the patient was taken and recorded at regular intervals, as was the exact time when signs and symptoms began to surface. Among the most common clinical manifestations seen was nystagmus, blurred vision, or diplopia; paresthesias in the lower extremities; hyperreflexia; spasticity; and muscle fatigue. Muscle fatigue was reported prior to the onset of upper motor neuron signs.

Based on the premise that led to the implementation of the Hot Bath Test Procedure as a diagnostic tool for patients with multiple sclerosis, heat is considered a contraindication. Therefore, if aquatic rehabilitation is considered, water temperature should not exceed 90°F. The ideal temperature should range between 88°F and 90°F.

The patient with MS will benefit from selected aquatic therapy interventions and from tailored aquatic programs of activities and exercises. If the patient is spastic, the DASI approach suggests the application of Bad Ragaz spasticity inhibiting patterns including the passive relaxation position. The passive trunk elongation with pelvic hold pattern might be very effective in decreasing lower extremity extensor tone by maintaining hip abduction. The DASI theory does not advocate the application of Bad Ragaz patterns that are meant to increase muscle strength as these might increase spasticity. Once a decrease in tone is noticed, the Watsu® basic flow sequence can be integrated into the plan of care. Watsu® movement sequences that particularly induce flexibility and enhance hypotonicity are very effective. These movement sequences include the bilateral repetitive flexion-extension, bilateral repetitive rotational flexion-extension, the unilateral ipsilateral lower extremity rotation, and the capture. Depending on the degree of efficacy obtained with the application of Watsu® Basic Flow, the therapist might consider integrating selected transitional flow sequences.

If the patient is ambulatory, Halliwick balance and weight-shifting activities could prove effective, particularly in cases of cerebellar involvement.

The therapist can also implement other shallow-water dynamic aquatic therapy activities and exercises. Such activities may include aquatic gait training with selected gait patterns such as forward gait, retrogait, and side-stepping gait. The modified side-stepping crab walk might help to improve coordination deficits in the patient with ataxia. Deep-water jogging using floatation devices will help with trunk stability and improve reciprocal motor activity. The therapist must monitor the patient during dynamic shallow and deep-water activities for the onset of muscle fatigue. If muscle fatigue develops, the activity should be discontinued and modified once the patient recovers.

Multiple Sclerosis Case Study

The following case utilizes the DASI pre-aquatic assessment form to present clinical findings, establish goals, and select the interventions that would best meet the established goals. A discussion of the case is provided to justify the selection of activities, techniques, and interventions and to suggest other potentially effective strategies in the clinical management of the patient with MS.

DASI
Diagnostic Aquatics Systems Integration — Pre-Aquatic Therapy Assessment

Patient Name: _____*Sally*_____ Date: _____

Dx: ____*Multiple Sclerosis*_____ Age: ____*50*_____

> **History/Problems/Complaints:** *This patient was diagnosed with multiple sclerosis three years ago. Her primary complaints are frequent episodes of muscle fatigue exacerbated by physical activity. Medication regime consists of Baclofen 10 mg TID and Clonopin .5 mg TID. Pt. denies any current bladder or bowel problems.*
> **Clinical Impression:** *Ataxia with Extensor LE Spasticity secondary to multiple sclerosis*

Musculoskeletal Assessment

Musculoskeletal Assessment		Manual Muscle Test		Range of Motion	
		Right	Left	Right	Left
Shoulder	Flexors	4-/5	4-/5	WFL	WFL
	Extensors	4-/5	4-/5	WFL	WFL
	Abductors	4-/5	4-/5	WFL	WFL
	Adductors	4-/5	4-/5	WFL	WFL
	External Rotators	4-/5	4-/5	WFL	WFL
	Internal Rotators	4-/5	4-/5	WFL	WFL
Elbow	Flexors	4-/5	4-/5	WFL	WFL
	Extensors	4-/5	4-/5	WFL	WFL
Forearm	Pronators	4-/5	4-/5	WFL	WFL
	Supinators	4-/5	4-/5	WFL	WFL
Wrist	Flexors	4-/5	4-/5	WFL	WFL
	Extensors	4-/5	4-/5	WFL	WFL
Finger	Flexors/Hand Grip	3/5	3/5	WFL	WFL
Hip	Flexors	3-/5	3-/5	WFL	WFL
	Extensors	2+/5	2+/5	WFL	WFL
	Abductors	2+/5	2+/5	WFL	WFL
	Adductors	3-/5	3-/5	WFL	WFL
	External Rotators	2-/5	2-/5	WFL	WFL
	Internal Rotators	3/5	3/5	WFL	WFL

Musculoskeletal Assessment		Manual Muscle Test		Range of Motion	
		Right	Left	Right	Left
Knee	Flexors	3-/5	3-/5	WFL	WFL
	Extensors	3-/5	3-/5	WFL	WFL
Ankle	Dorsiflexors	2-/5	2-/5	WFL	WFL
	Plantar Flexors	3/5	3/5	WFL	WFL
Foot	Invertors	3/5	3/5	WFL	WFL
	Evertors	3-/5	3-/5	WFL	WFL

Musculoskeletal Assessment		ROM	MMT
Spine	Cervical Flexion	WFL	4-/5
	Cervical Extension	WFL	4-/5
	Cervical Lateral Flexion (right)	WFL	4-/5
	Cervical Lateral Flexion (left)	WFL	4-/5
	Cervical Rotation (right)	WFL	4-/5
	Cervical Rotation (left)	WFL	4-/5
	Lumbar Flexion	WFL	5/5
	Lumbar Extension	WFL	5/5
	Lumbar Lateral Flexion (right)	WFL	5/5
	Lumbar Lateral Flexion (left)	WFL	5/5

Evidence of Edema? ☐ Yes ■ No

Girth Anatomical Landmark: ____ ■ Not Applicable		
Right: _____inch(es)	Left: _____ inch(es)	

Leg-Length Discrepancy? ☐ Yes ■ No
Approximate Discrepancy: _____ inch(es)

Musculoskeletal Assessment (continued)

Posture

Posture	❑ Normal Alignment ■ Postural Deviations Explain *forward head; scoliosis with right convexity*

Spasmodic Activity

❑ No evidence of muscle spasms	**Grade**			
■ Not applicable	**1**	**2**	**3**	**4**

	Muscles				
Spasmodic Activity					

Cardiopulmonary Assessment

Cardiopulmonary Assessment

Lungs	■ Clear to Auscultation ❑ Abnormal Breath Sounds ❑ Adventitious Breath Sounds ■ Resonant Chest to Mediate Percussion ❑ Other: ❑ Bibasilar Thoracic Asymmetry RR: _____ ■ Normal ❑ Dyspnea ❑ Other:
Cardiac	■ Normal S1 Other: ■ Normal S2 ❑ Split S1 ❑ Split S2 ❑ S3 ❑ S4 ❑ Murmur ❑ Ejection Click HR: *70* BP: *118/78*

Neurological Assessment

Neurologic Assessment

Superficial Sensation	❑ Intact **Explain** ■ Impaired *Anterior aspects of bilateral thighs; lateral aspect of bilateral legs; dorsum and plantar surface of feet bilaterally*
Coordination	❑ Intact **Explain** ■ Impaired ❑ Intention Tremors *BLE exhibiting ataxia*
Proprioception	❑ Intact **Explain** ■ Impaired *Impaired in both lower extremities*
Deep Tendon Reflexes	❑ Intact **Explain** ■ Diminished *bilateral patellar (almost areflexic) and Achilles tendon reflexes* ❑ Hyperactive _____
Balance	Static ❑ Intact ■ Impaired Dynamic ❑ Intact ■ Impaired

Pain	No Pain Intolerable Pain 0 1 ■ 3 4 5 6 7 8 9 10 *Bilateral Triceps Surae particularly at night with spasticity episodes*
Tone	❑ Normal ■ Hypertonia / Spasticity *Moderate extensor spasticity of BLE's; bilateral clonus* ❑ Hypotonia / Flaccidity ❑ Cogwheel Rigidity ❑ Contractures

		Check the Appropriate Box		
		Pos	Neg	N/A
Other Neurologic Test Results	SLR Test	❑	❑	■
	Neural Tension	❑	❑	■
		Ulnar	Radial	Median
	Fabere Sign	❑	❑	■
	Compression Test	❑	❑	■
	Distraction Stretch	❑	❑	■
	Vertebral Artery Test	❑	❑	■
	Alar Ligament Test	❑	❑	■
	Vertebral Glide Test	❑	❑	■
	Babinski Sign	■	❑	❑
	Romberg's Test	■	❑	❑
	Other	■	❑	❑
	Positive clonus on bilateral ankles/feet			

Functional Assessment

Mobility		
Gait Analysis		■ Ambulatory ❑ Non-Ambulatory Explain: *pt. ambulates with KAFO using reciprocal walker but additionally uses electric wheelchair with hand held knob control when experiencing increased fatigue or spasticity with pain* ■ Assistive Device: *KAFO; electrically powered wheelchair with hand control; Reciprocal walker* Weight Bearing: ■ FWB ❑ PWB ❑ NWB ❑ No significant gait deviations noted. ■ Gait Deviations: *bilateral hip hiking on midswing with increased hip and knee flexion; decreased heel strike on early stance* ■ Abnormal Gait *Steppage gait*
Bed Mobility		❑ Independent ■ Requires assistance ❑ max ❑ mod ■ min
Transfers		❑ Independent ■ Requires assistance ❑ max ■ mod ❑ min
Body Mechanics		■ Not tested ❑ Uses proper body mechanics when lifting, carrying, sitting, and lying down ❑ Does not use proper body mechanics when lifting, carrying, and lying down ❑ Needs further instruction and practice

Goals

■ Improve endurance
■ Improve balance
❑ Improve spinal mobility
■ Promote relaxation
❑ Improve breathing patterns
_____

❑ Decrease pain
_____

■ Increase muscle strength
on muscle groups with documented weakness
❑ Increase joint range and flexibility
_____

■ Improve gait pattern
■ Improve coordination and proprioception
❑ Reduce muscle fatigue
❑ Decrease edema and inflammation
_____

■ Improve postural alignment
❑ Improve circulation
■ Improve motor control
■ Inhibit spasticity/hypertonicity
BLE's as documented
❑ Resolution of muscle spasms: _____
_____

Plan of Care

Frequency: __3__ times per week for _4_ weeks

Bad Ragaz	■ Passive Relaxation ❑ Passive Pelvic Tilts ■ Pre-Gait ❑ Isotonic #1 ❑ Isotonic #2 ❑ Isometric ❑ Pre-Weight-Bearing ■ Tone Inhibition ■ Passive Trunk Elongation/Knee Hold ■ Passive Trunk Elongation/Pelvic Hold ❑ Passive Trunk Elongation/Thoracic Hold ■ Unilateral Upper Extremity ■ Bilateral Upper Extremity ❑ Prone Unilateral Upper Extremity ■ Unilateral Lower Extremity ❑ Bilateral Lower Extremity ■ Bilateral Symmetrical Lower Extremity #1 ❑ Bilateral Symmetrical Lower Extremity #2 ❑ Bilateral Reciprocal Lower Extremity ❑ Other:
Halliwick	■ Phase I Adjustment ■ Phase II Rotational Activities ❑ Turbulent Gliding ❑ Balance Training/Kangaroo Jumps ■ Balance Training/Weight Shifting ❑ Other: _____

Cardiaquatics	❑ Level I Sequences: _____ Activities: ____
	❑ Level II Sequences: _____ Activities: ____
	❑ Level III Sequences: _____ Activities: ____
	❑ Level IV
	    ❑ Phase 1 ❑ Phase 2 ❑ Phase 3 ❑ All
	    ❑ Selected Sequences:

Other	❑ Applied Myofascial Release ❑ Deep Friction Massage ❑ Applied Joint Mobilization/Distraction ❑ Applied Spinal Mobilization/Distraction ❑ Applied Joint Approximation ❑ Applied Feldenkrais ❑ Applied Lymphatic Drainage ■ Watsu/Basic Flow ■ Watsu/Transitional Flow ❑ Clinical Wassertanzen I ❑ Clinical Wassertanzen II ❑ Clinical Wassertanzen III ❑ Applied Aquatic Craniosacral Therapy ❑ Trigger Point Therapy ❑ Ai Chi: _____ ❑ Spinal/Trunk Stabilization Protocol: _____ ❑ Thoracic Outlet Syndrome Protocol: _____ ❑ Other: _____

Functional / Goal Specific Aquatic Therapy Activities and Exercises

■ Gait Training (<u>Forward</u>/Backward) Laps: _3____
❑ Stair Climbing x _____
❑ Bicycling Reps: _____
❑ Prone Activities Min _____
■ Aquajogging Laps: _1-2__
❑ Heel Cord Stretch
❑ Iliopsoas Stretch
❑ Piriformis Stretch
❑ TFL Stretch
❑ IT Band Stretch
❑ Hip Add Stretch
❑ Stork Stand
❑ Front to Back Weight Shifting
❑ Side to Side Weight Shifting
❑ Heel Raises Reps: _____
❑ Four-Corner Pivot Reps: ____

■ Side-Stepping Laps: _3____
❑ Cross Over Stepping Laps: _____
❑ Deep-Water Stride Jump Reps: ____
❑ Deep-Water Jogging (fwd/retro): _____ min.
❑ Deep-Water Groin Stretch
❑ Knee to Chest Reps: _____
❑ Closed Kinematic Chain Exercises
❑ Deep-Water Double Knee Lifts Reps: _____
❑ Wall Slide Reps: ____
❑ Pelvic Tilts Reps: ___
❑ Supine Kicks Reps:____
❑ Deep-Water Spinal Traction in Vertical Suspension
   (_____ lbs. x _____ min.)
❑ Resistive Exercises:
■ Other: _Side-Stepping Crab Walk x 3 laps with Halliwick short/long arm hold_

Aquatic Work Conditioning

❑ Resistive Forward/Retro Gait x _____ laps
❑ Deep-Water Jogging (fwd/retro) x _____ min.
❑ Tethered Jogging # ____ x _____ min.
❑ Swimming: _____laps/min

❑ Other:_____

Equipment Used

■ Bodyfit® Collar
❑ Floatation Vest
❑ Tire Tube
■ Floatation Pelvic Belt
❑ Fins
❑ Snorkel Mask
❑ Snorkel Tube
■ Ankle Floats
❑ Aqua-Dumbbells

❑ AquaJogger
❑ Graduated-Resistance Paddles
❑ Hydrotone Boots
❑ Hoola Hoop
❑ Resistance Cord
❑ Thera-Band®
❑ Aquakinetic Machines
❑ Boards
■ Floatation Noodle

❑ Hydrotone Dumbbells
❑ Weights: _____
■ Bad Ragaz Floatation Rings
❑ Swim Bar
❑ Recumbent Bicycle
❑ Underwater Treadmill
❑ Halliwick Blow Balls
■ Other: _Bilateral KAFOs for pool therapy use only_

Adjunct Therapy

■ Not Applicable

❑ Whirlpool: ____ min. (spa)

❑ Patient Education

❑ Posture and Body Mechanics

❑ Home Exercise Program

❑ Other:_____

Land Based Therapy Treatments

❑ Not Applicable

Frequency: _____ times per week
          for _____ weeks
❑ US: _____
❑ ES: _____

❑ HP's: _____
❑ Massage: _____
❑ Piriformis Release
❑ Therapeutic Exercises (specify):

❑ Paraffin Bath:

■ Cryotherapy: _Ice massage to hip and knee extensors, ankle plantar flexors as needed to decrease spasticity prior to pool session_
❑ Joint Mobilization:
❑ Other:

Comments:

_____   _____
Signature & Credentials of Therapist   Date

Discussion

Sally is a female patient with MS who remains active despite her condition. At the time of her referral for aquatic therapy services she was in remission. Sometimes she plateaus in a long-term remission secondary to the effects of Baclofen and Clonopin, which decrease spasticity and the incidence of pain from spastic nocturnal episodes.

Her primary clinical problems are intermittent episodes of extensor hypertonicity interfering with daily activities. She exhibits a steppage gait because of weakness of the flexor musculature in the lower extremities. Her disease has progressed over a period of three years even though she experiences frequent remissions that may last several months before the onset of a relapse.

This patient will benefit from any intervention directed towards inhibiting spasticity. Consequently, selected Bad Ragaz patterns where the hip is flexed and externally rotated or where the knees are flexed will be conducive to this goal. Besides the Bad Ragaz tone inhibition pattern, the passive trunk elongation patterns with pelvic and knee hold would also serve the same purpose in addition to maintaining range of motion. The same is true of the bilateral symmetrical lower extremity #1 pattern. Since the upper extremities are not extensively affected, maintenance of range of motion and strength should be emphasized with the application of Bad Ragaz upper extremity patterns.

Since the patient presents with balance and coordination deficits, Halliwick Phase I techniques, particularly the integration of adapted balance activities, should be practiced. Once there is evidence of improved trunk control and balance, Phase II rotation activities in shallow or deep water may be integrated. If these are performed in deep water, floatation equipment will be needed, as will the guidance, contact guarding, and assistance of the therapist. Other dynamic shallow-water activities with applied Halliwick concepts and principles include gait training. The therapist should consider guarding the patient through the application of the Halliwick short- or long-arm hold technique. The crab walk serves various purposes. First, the position of the patient in this activity will be conducive to inhibition of spasticity. Second, this activity is also meant to improve dynamic balance. Third, it works on the improvement of gait deficits. For gait training purposes, it might be helpful to have an additional KAFO to be used for aquatic therapy sessions exclusively.

CHAPTER 11

MUSCULOSKELETAL APPLICATIONS

Fibromyalgia

Once called fibrositis, fibromyalgia has been defined as a chronic, complex condition causing widespread pain and fatigue in muscles, tendons, and ligaments. Although its etiology is unknown, stress, physical trauma, infections, and emotional instability have been identified as predisposing factors that trigger the onset of symptoms.

Muscle pain is the primary symptom in patients diagnosed with fibromyalgia syndrome (FMS). Patients generally report burning pain of a gradual or abrupt onset. This pain is the result of muscle microtrauma, which leads to localized inflammatory reactions and increased incidence of spasmodic activity. The incidence of widespread muscle spasms in the patient with FMS elicits a spasm-pain-spasm cycle.

A disruption of stage IV non-REM (non-rapid eye movement) sleep is another characteristic manifestation of FMS. Loss of non-REM sleep generally leads to fatigue, inactivity, and deconditioning; increasing stress levels; and tension resulting in higher levels of spasmodic activity and muscle microtrauma. Consequently, the abnormal sleep pattern of alpha non-REM is related to the degree and extent of stiffness and achiness.

In the diagnostic process, the American College of Rheumatology identifies key "trigger points" in the patient suspected of having FMS (Figure 213). I define "trigger points" as tender or pain-sensitive areas. If the patient presents evidence of having at least eleven of the eighteen tender points when pressure is applied upon palpation, the diagnosis is a positive one. These "trigger points" are:

1. bilateral suboccipital insertions (2)
2. intertransverse spaces between C5 and C7 (4)

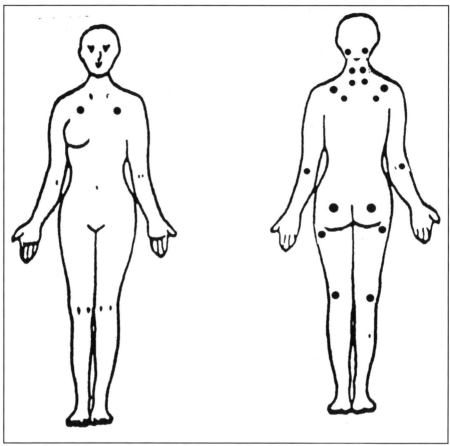

Figure 213: Trigger points in the fibromyalgia patient.

3. midpoint of bilateral upper trape-zius (2)
4. bilateral origins of the supraspina-tus near the medial border of the spine of the scapula (2)
5. bilateral second costochondral junction (2)
6. lateral epicondyles bilaterally (2)
7. bilateral gluteus maximus and piriformis (2)
8. bilateral greater trochanters posteri-orly (2)
9. medial aspect of the knee near the pes anserinus and posterior towards the popliteal fat pad (2).

The incidence of FMS is most prevalent in women between the ages of 20 and 50. Frequent headaches and migraines are reported by many patients with FMS secondary to suboccipital, cervical, and scapular involvement. In some cases, TMJ problems have been reported. Other described systemic manifestations include irritable bowel syndrome and vestibular problems that may be accompanied by tinnitus.

Muscle relaxants such as Flexeril or Elavil have proven effective in the pharmacotherapeutic management of patients with FMS. These drugs boost the levels of serotonin and norepineph-rine, thereby improving circadian rhythms and decreasing the onset and severity of muscle spasms. The same is true of selected antidepressants such as amytriptiline.

Aquatic rehabilitation has also been remarkably successful in relieving identified clinical problems in the patient with FMS. A combination of thermotherapeutic and hydrotherapeutic effects are responsible for this success. However, the application of selected specialized interventions such as Watsu® and the Clinical Wassertanzen Protocol has further enhanced the attainment of established goals and objectives in patients with fibromyalgia.

A Pilot Single-Case Study on the Effects of the Clinical Wassertanzen Protocol on a Patient with Fibromyalgia

In April 1999, I completed a single baseline research study on a patient with fibromyalgia with the intent to prove that the Clinical Wassertanzen Protocol was an effective intervention in relieving symptoms and improving the overall quality of life in these patients. The patient studied was a forty-nine-year-old female who reported a high stress level administrative job. Her diagnosis was made in November 1998. Prior to considering the

application of Clinical Wassertanzen as the primary treatment intervention, the patient was treated with other aquatic and land therapy techniques.

Methodology and Procedure

Once the pre-aquatic assessment was completed, an informed consent was signed by the patient affirming that she fully agreed to participate in the study. The patient was also comprehensively oriented and instructed in the three phases of this aquatic therapy intervention with emphasis on instruction and practice in the three phases of breathing control.

Once the study began, the patient was treated twice a week for a period of three weeks. Each treatment consisted of a forty-five minute session where the Clinical Wassertanzen Protocol was applied. The first session emphasized the first two phases of the protocol. However, due to the patient's increased tolerance to submersions, subsequent sessions focused on the second and third phases of the protocol.

The evaluation criteria featured three measured target behaviors. These were pain levels, sleep pattern, and spasmodic activity. Pain levels were measured using the Numeric Pain

Table 3: Sleep Pattern Scale

Scale	Sleep Percentage	Description
4	100%	Uninterrupted sleep activity; slept all night without interruptions.
3	75%	Occasional interruptions in sleep pattern; slept most of the night with only a couple of interruptions.
2	50%	Able to sleep half the night but could not sleep the first or second half due to pain and discomfort.
1	25%	Only able to sleep for a couple of hours at a time; woke up every two hours with pain and discomfort.
0	0%	Unable to sleep the entire night due to pain and discomfort.
© 2004 Luis Vargas		

Table 4: Maneuvers for fibromyalgia experiment.

Phase II	• Lateral sacral glides • Soft tissue and myofascial releases (ipsilateral, contralateral, and paraspinal • Trigger point releases • Cervical spine distraction • Cradled rocking
Phase III	• Passive full body flexion • Passive maneuvers of the pelvic belt musculature (proximal and distal hold) • Pelvic and spine rotations • Prone spine snaking maneuver • Thoracolumbar flexion-extension • Scapulohumeral distraction • Scapulothoracic mobilization • Thoracodorsal maneuver • Lumbopelvic and sacroiliac stabilization

Scale. This scale, which is featured in the DASI Pre-Aquatic Assessment discussed in Chapter 2 as the pain evaluation instrument, describes the highest recorded level of pain as a "10" with the lowest being a "0," which represents no pain.

I designed a sleep pattern scale that objectively measured sleep activity (Table 3). The sleep pattern scale consisted of five ratings. A rating of "4" indicated uninterrupted sleep throughout the night. Progressively, the rating

dropped consistent with deterioration in sleep activity to "0."

Finally, evidence of spasmodic activity was determined through manual examination, applying the trigger point test along with surface anatomy techniques, to identify and grade muscle spasms present in any of the eighteen pain-sensitive areas. The DASI Spasmodic Activity Grading (SAG) Scale, which is discussed in Chapter 2, was the instrument used to measure the presence, severity, and extent of muscle

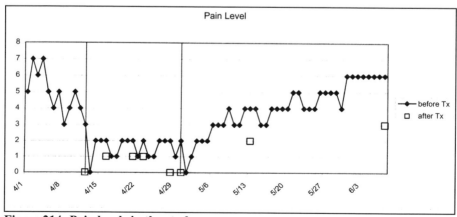

Figure 214: Pain levels in the study.

spasms, which ranged from "0" to "4." For instance, a grade of "0" would indicate no spasmodic activity whereas a grade of "4" suggested widespread excessive tension of soft tissue structures from origin to insertion.

All three target behaviors were recorded before and after each Clinical Wassertanzen session. The applied maneuvers used are listed in Table 4.

Data Analysis

Visual analysis and the Friedman two-way analysis of variance by rank were the primary instruments used in the analysis of collected data.

In the visual analysis of pain level (Figure 214), the period from April 1st to April 12th is the baseline. This represents the period of time when the patient was not receiving Clinical Wassertanzen sessions. Nevertheless, the patient was asked to record her pain levels prior to the beginning of Clinical Wassertanzen for a two-week period. The intervention phase in visual analysis terminology marks the period from April 12th through April 30th (shown between the vertical bars). The maintenance phase begins on May 1st and extends through June 7th. The boxes

(□) represent the pain levels reported by the patient after the Clinical Wassertanzen session. Notice that there was a significant reduction of pain level progressively from the first to the last treatment. This improvement remained constant at a much lower level than what was recorded in the baseline section. This clearly demonstrates that the residual therapeutic effects were still present upon the conclusion of the study.

A similar trend in improvement resulting from the therapeutic effect is noticed in the analysis of sleep pattern (Figure 215). The baseline section reveals disrupted sleep activity with a significant increase in uninterrupted sleep during the intervention phase. Notice that the patient once again demonstrated high levels of interrupted sleep activity after the intervention phase concluded. However, she did report an improvement on two occasions during the maintenance phase. The rationale for the two treatments that were administered during the maintenance phase was to establish a continuum and prevalence of the therapeutic effects once the intervention phase ended. This rationale also applies

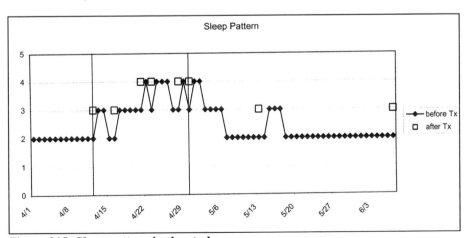

Figure 215: Sleep pattern in the study.

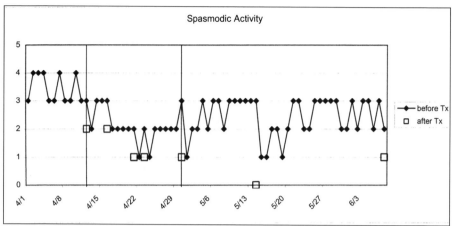

Figure 216: Degree of spasmodic activity in the study.

to the other two measured target behaviors.

Spasmodic activity was identified in the upper trapezius, splenii, levator scapulae, rhomboids, and infraspinatus muscles. The graph (Figure 216) shows a high incidence of muscle spasms in the baseline section followed by a considerable decrease throughout the intervention and maintenance phases, which remained at a plateau thereafter as compared to the baseline data.

Results

In order to determine whether or not this particular aquatic therapy intervention had a significant effect in decreasing pain levels, improving sleep patterns, and resolving muscle spasms, a pre- and post-measurement of each target behavior was recorded in every treatment session. Based on the results obtained (Table 5), I failed to reject the

true hypothesis but yet rejected the null.

Through the use of the Friedman Two-Way Analysis of Variance by rank instrument for data analysis, the calculated value is noticeably higher than the critical value on all three target behaviors. The calculated value results strongly support the hypothesis.

Limitations and Assumptions

The primary limitation in this study was the lack of a large enough sample of the population. However, having proven the hypothesis in this single case design, it could set the stage for yet another study that could involve a much larger population sample.

Conclusion

As reported by the patient, the applied maneuvers that were particularly effective in this case were the prone spine snaking, scapulothoracic mobili-

Table 5: Statistical summary of study

1. Pain Level:	$X_r^2 = 8$
for k=3, n=8, critical value at $X_r^2 = 6.250$ at $\alpha = .05$	
2. Sleep Pattern:	$X_r^2 = 8$
for k=3, n=8, critical value at $X_r^2 = 6.250$ at $\alpha = .05$	
3. Spasmodic Activity:	$X_r^2 = 8$
for k=3, n=8, critical value at $X_r^2 = 6.250$ at $\alpha = .05$	

zation with soft tissue release, scapulo-humeral distraction, and the trigger point releases followed by cervical distraction. The patient rapidly gained proficiency in the three phases of breathing control achieving a submersion tolerance of forty-five seconds to one minute.

Clinical Wassertanzen is an advanced level aquatic therapy intervention. It is important to mention that not every patient with FMS is a candidate for this therapeutic procedure. The effects are powerful but multiple factors must be taken into consideration. The circumstances surrounding each case must be carefully analyzed and a meticulous pre-aquatic evaluation must be completed. The evaluation must include a comprehensive interview in order to provide the therapist with foresight on the patient's expected tolerance to submersions. Should the patient not be an ideal candidate for Clinical Wassertanzen, Watsu® is an excellent alternative intervention for patients with fibromyalgia. The therapist should exercise caution in the selection of aquatic therapy activities because these might increase the chances of micro-traumatizing the muscle fiber and eliciting the syndrome. Aquatic therapy for the patient with fibromyalgia should focus on the two "Rs," relaxation and release.

Low Back Pain

Low back pain is a term used to describe a wide range of neurological and/or musculoskeletal manifestations, which result from injury to the spine and its associated soft and connective tissue structures. It figures among the most commonly treated diagnoses in aquatic rehabilitation.

Radiculopathies are a common cause of low back pain. The spinal root as it exits through the intervertebral foramen is compressed, leading to a clinical picture of symptoms and signs that follow the anatomical distribution of the compressed nerve root. This compression can be caused by a herniated intervertebral disc, a rotated vertebra, infections, malignancy, or neurological disease affecting the spinal cord and nerves.

Although it might occur at any level of the vertebral column, the incidence is greater in the lumbar region. Lumbar radiculopathies are most often seen as a result of herniated discs. The intervertebral disc rests between the bodies of the vertebrae forming the anterior intervertebral joint. This structure consists of an outer fibrocartilaginous ring called the annulus fibrosus and an inner gelatinous substance known as the nucleus pulposus. It acts as a shock absorber for axial forces that are transmitted to this area. When the axial forces are excessive, a herniation of the nucleus pulposus (HNP) occurs. Most frequently HNPs happen postero-laterally. The result is the onset of radicular neuralgia following the path of the major constituents of the lumbosacral plexus. Any of the nerves that form the lumbosacral plexus can be affected. Sometimes the clinical findings suggest multiple nerve involvement. However, the sciatic nerve is often the most affected leading to a number of clinical manifestations that are collectively referred to as sciatica.

Low back pain can be both localized and radiated. Localized pain is identified around the area of herniation or radiculitis with increased spasmodic activity and tenderness in the adjacent paraspinal region. Radiated pain follows the anatomical pathway of the compressed nerve root or roots ending with motor and sensory manifestations in the terminal nerve or nerves. A combination of the two is not uncommon. Therefore, the patient will report high levels of pain at the time of the pre-aquatic assessment. If a patient with low back pain reports severe pain that renders him unable to perform weight-bearing activities even in shallow water, it is strongly advised to begin with deep-water dynamic activities. Based on my experience, an effective strategy in relieving pain levels is to place a floatation belt or vest on the patient and allow him to vertically suspend himself in deep water for approximately twenty minutes. Five to ten pound cuff weights are placed around both ankles. The technique is known as deep-water, vertical suspension traction and is quite effective in decreasing pain that interferes with the patient's treatment. This technique is later complemented with the integration of deep-water jogging activities.

Patients with low back pain will exhibit postural deviations that are the consequence of their constant guarding against the pain. This will also lead to widespread spasmodic activity in the paraspinal region and around the gluteal area. A posturally rotated pelvis is one of the signs of malalignment identified during the assessment. Secondary to this occurrence, a surface anatomy examination with trigger point tests will indicate a severely spasmodic piriformis muscle with increased tenderness in the area. Should this be the case, the primary objective should focus on releasing the piriformis tightness. A tight piriformis muscle causes pressure on the trunk of the sciatic nerve, which courses directly under this muscle, intensifying the motor and sensory manifestations in the soft tissue distal to

this compression. This is called the Piriformis Syndrome. Releasing a tight piriformis can be accomplished through several techniques:

1. Active piriformis stretch in shallow water
2. A land-based passive piriformis release applying the trigger point release technique followed by whirlpool therapy
3. The application of land-based therapeutic massage focusing on pétrissage, effleurage, and deep cross-friction to the gluteal region with emphasis on the piriformis muscle
4. The application of thermotherapeutic land-based modalities such as ultrasound
5. Selected Watsu® basic and transitional flow sequences such as:
   a. the bilateral repetitive lower extremity rotational flexor-extensor pattern
   b. the unilateral hip and knee flexion with rotation pattern
   c. the contralateral passive stretch technique to the shoulder adductors, shoulder flexors, hip extensors, and hip adductors
   d. the sustained trunk and lateral thigh stretch technique
   e. the full range contralateral hip flexion with gluteal and lumbar soft tissue stretch.

A combination of manual land-based release techniques and integrated aquatic interventions should be considered for optimal results. The therapist should wear gloves and should use a moisturizing lotion when applying therapeutic massage or land-based release techniques. Penetrating ointments containing menthol can also be used but caution must be taken to prevent contact with sensitive tissues.

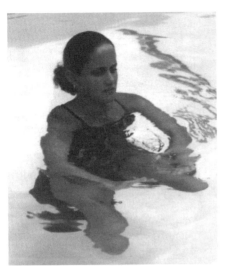

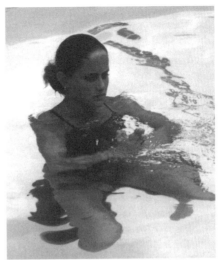

Figure 217: Stage II pelvic and trunk stabilization in deep water using the kick board...

Figure 218: ...to move into the prayer position.

Menthol-based penetrating ointments might be more effective when treating the lumbar, scapular, or cervical regions.

Another land-based pre-aquatic technique effectively used to passively release the piriformis muscle involves placing the patient in the prone position on the treatment table with the affected leg off the edge of the table. The knee is flexed, either resting on a chair or on another clinician's thigh or hand. This position can be modified based on the patient's tolerance level. An alternate position consists of placing the patient in the prone position on the treatment table with a pillow under the hips and abdomen, and a towel roll under the ankles. If at all possible, a massage table should be used. This table has an attachment for the face allowing the patient to be more comfortable during the technique. The therapist uses his elbow, his knuckles, or his thumb as a pressure and trigger point release medium. Pressure is applied at the point of highest spasmodic activity. If another clinician is not available to assist, the patient may be positioned prone one quarter of a turn towards side-lying with the knee flexed on the table. This technique proves to be quite painful for the patient before some relief is experienced. The patient should be draped adequately for the procedure and privacy should be observed. Whirlpool therapy should be administered for five to ten minutes following the release. Whirlpool therapy is contraindicated if the patient has a history of high blood pressure or any cardiac condition. In that case, continuing with deep-water activities such as vertical suspension with traction or deep-water jogging might prove more appropriate.

As pain lessens and the patient's ability to perform activities in shallow and deep water improves, the integration of trunk stability activities in both shallow and deep water can be added as a supplement to the aquatic care. The use of floatation equipment should be avoided if a trunk stability protocol is implemented. The sequence of deep-water activities featured in the trunk stability protocol is as follows:

Stage I: Swim Bar Activities

1. Patient stands on a swim bar with arms abducted at 90°; a swim bar can be held on each hand to maintain the position.
2. Patient stands on a swim bar with hands clasped together in prayer position.

Stage II: Kick Board Activities

1. Patient sits on the board with arms crossed over shoulders
2. Patient sits on the board with hands clasped together in prayer position (Figure 217 and Figure 218).
3. Patient stands on the board with a rubber ball pressed between both knees; arms abducted.
4. Patient stand on the board maintaining an upright posture; hands clasped together in prayer position.

Another group of patients that fall in this category are patients who have undergone surgical intervention for a spine condition. Spinal surgical procedures that may be treated by aquatic therapy include laminectomies, discectomies, and spinal fusions. The most important consideration to keep in mind with patients who have had spinal surgical procedures, particularly with spinal fusions, is the fixed and limited spinal joint range that remains after the surgery. Therefore, interventions that promote movement and passive stretch in the soft and connective tissue structures of the spine and pelvis are contraindicated. However, patients can perform selected shallow and deepwater dynamic activities. Flexion of the hips in excess of 90° should be avoided.

DASI
Diagnostic Aquatics Systems Integration — Pre-Aquatic Therapy Assessment

Patient Name: _____*Tom*_____   Date: _____

Dx: ___*Lumbar radiculopathy secondary to L3-L4 herniation*___   Age: ___*33*_____

History/Problems/Complaints: *Pt. sustained a work-related injury to his low back while lifting a heavy steel bar resulting in L3-L4, L5-S1 HNP with residual lumbago and sciatica. He is being treated medically through worker's compensation with anti-inflammatory and pain relief medications. Pt. was recently treated unsuccessfully with land-based therapy. TENS was applied but only offered temporary symptomatic relief. He is now referred to aquatic therapy for evaluation and treatment.*
Clinical Impression: *Low back pain and piriformis syndrome with lumbar radiculopathy*

Musculoskeletal Assessment

Musculoskeletal Assessment		Manual Muscle Test		Range of Motion	
		Right	Left	Right	Left
Shoulder	Flexors	4+/5	4+/5	WFL	WFL
	Extensors	4+/5	4+/5	WFL	WFL
	Abductors	4+/5	4+/5	WFL	WFL
	Adductors	4+/5	4+/5	WFL	WFL
	External Rotators	4+/5	4+/5	WFL	WFL
	Internal Rotators	4+/5	4+/5	WFL	WFL
Elbow	Flexors	4+/5	4+/5	WFL	WFL
	Extensors	4/5	4/5	WFL	WFL
Forearm	Pronators	5/5	5/5	WFL	WFL
	Supinators	5/5	5/5	WFL	WFL
Wrist	Flexors	5/5	5/5	WFL	WFL
	Extensors	4+/5	4+/5	WFL	WFL
Finger	Flexors/Hand Grip	4+/5	4+/5	WFL	WFL
Hip	Flexors	3+/5	4-/5	WFL	WFL
	Extensors	3/5	4-/5	5°	10°
	Abductors	3/5	4-/5	WFL	WFL
	Adductors	4/5	4+/5	WFL	WFL
	External Rotators	3/5	3+/5	WFL	WFL
	Internal Rotators	3/5	3+/5	20°	WFL

Musculoskeletal Assessment		Manual Muscle Test		Range of Motion	
		Right	Left	Right	Left
Knee	Flexors	3/5	4-/5	WFL	WFL
	Extensors	4/5	4/5	WFL	WFL
Ankle	Dorsiflexors	4/5	4/5	WFL	WFL
	Plantar Flexors	4+/5	4+/5	WFL	WFL
Foot	Invertors	4+/5	4+/5	WFL	WFL
	Evertors	4+/5	4+/5	WFL	WFL

Musculoskeletal Assessment		ROM	MMT
Spine	Cervical Flexion	WFL	4/5
	Cervical Extension	WFL	4-/5
	Cervical Lateral Flexion (right)	WFL	4/5
	Cervical Lateral Flexion (left)	WFL	4/5
	Cervical Rotation (right)	WFL	4/5
	Cervical Rotation (left)	WFL	4/5
	Lumbar Flexion	5°	4/5
	Lumbar Extension	0°	4/5
	Lumbar Lateral Flexion (right)	0°	4/5
	Lumbar Lateral Flexion (left)	12°	4/5

Evidence of Edema?   ❏ Yes   ■ No

Girth Anatomical Landmark: _____ ■ Not Applicable

Right:	_____inch(es)	Left:	_____ inch(es)

Leg-Length Discrepancy?   ❏ Yes   ■ No
Approximate Discrepancy: _____ inch(es)

Cardiopulmonary Assessment

Musculoskeletal Assessment (continued)

Posture

Posture	❐ Normal Alignment ■ Postural Deviations Explain *Forward head, kyphoscoliosis with right convexity, asymmetrical hip level rt. > lt., ant. rotated rt. pelvis*

Spasmodic Activity

❐ No evidence of muscle spasms ❐ Not applicable	Grade			
	1	**2**	**3**	**4**

	Muscles				
Spasmodic Activity	*rt. longissimus and spinalis*				■
	lt. longissimus and spinalis			■	
	rt. piriformis				■
	lt. piriformis			■	

Cardiopulmonary Assessment	
Lungs	■ Clear to Auscultation ❐ Abnormal Breath Sounds ❐ Adventitious Breath Sounds ❐ Resonant Chest to Mediate Percussion ❐ Other: ❐ Bibasilar Thoracic Asymmetry RR: *16/min* ■ Normal ❐ Dyspnea ■ Other: *Symmetrical thoracic excursions bilaterally*
Cardiac	■ Normal S1　　　Other: ■ Normal S2 ❐ Split S1 ❐ Split S2 ❐ S3 ❐ S4 ❐ Murmur ❐ Ejection Click HR: *84* BP: *128/80*

Neurological Assessment

Neurologic Assessment	
Superficial Sensation	❐ Intact　　　　　**Explain** ■ Impaired
Coordination	■ Intact　　　　　**Explain** ❐ Impaired ❐ Intention Tremors
Proprioception	■ Intact　　　　　**Explain** ❐ Impaired
Deep Tendon Reflexes	■ Intact　　　　　**Explain** ❐ Diminished _____ ❐ Hyperactive _____
Balance	Static　■ Intact　❐ Impaired Dynamic　■ Intact　❐ Impaired

Pain	No Pain　　　　　　Intolerable Pain 0　1　2　3　4　5　6　7　■　9　10 *bilateral lumbar regions and bilateral gluteal regions but > in rt. with radiation to post aspect of RLE*
Tone	■ Normal ❐ Hypertonia / Spasticity ❐ Hypotonia / Flaccidity ❐ Cogwheel Rigidity ❐ Contractures

Other Neurologic Test Results	Check the Appropriate Box		
	Pos	Neg	N/A
SLR Test	■	❐	❐
Neural Tension	❐	❐	■
Ulnar　Radial　Median			
Fabere Sign	■	❐	❐
Compression Test	❐	■	❐
Distraction Stretch	❐	❐	■
Vertebral Artery Test	❐	■	❐
Alar Ligament Test	❐	❐	■
Vertebral Glide Test	■	❐	❐
Babinski Sign	❐	❐	■
Romberg's Test	❐	❐	■
Other	■	❐	❐
positive Fabere bilaterally; positive vertebral glide on lumbar region			

Functional Assessment

Mobility

Gait Analysis	■ Ambulatory ❏ Non-Ambulatory Explain: ❏ Assistive Device: Weight Bearing: ■ FWB ❏ PWB ❏ NWB ❏ No significant gait deviations noted. ❏ Gait Deviations: ■ Abnormal Gait *antalgic gait secondary to pain and clinical manifestations*
Bed Mobility	■ Independent ❏ Requires assistance ❏ max ❏ mod ❏ min
Transfers	■ Independent ❏ Requires assistance ❏ max ❏ mod ❏ min
Body Mechanics	❏ Not tested ❏ Uses proper body mechanics when lifting, carrying, sitting, and lying down ■ Does not use proper body mechanics when lifting, carrying, and lying down ■ Needs further instruction and practice

Goals

■ Improve endurance
❏ Improve balance
■ Improve spinal mobility
❏ Promote relaxation
❏ Improve breathing patterns

■ Decrease pain
as documented
■ Increase muscle strength
in areas of weakness as documented
■ Increase joint range and flexibility
in areas with limitations as documented
■ Improve gait pattern
❏ Improve coordination and proprioception
❏ Reduce muscle fatigue
❏ Decrease edema and inflammation

■ Improve postural alignment
❏ Improve circulation
❏ Improve motor control
❏ Inhibit spasticity/hypertonicity

■ Resolution of muscle spasms: *in areas of increased spasmodic activity as documented*

Plan of Care

Frequency: _3_ times per week for _6_ weeks

Bad Ragaz	■ Passive Relaxation ■ Passive Pelvic Tilts ❏ Pre-Gait ❏ Isotonic #1 ❏ Isotonic #2 ❏ Isometric ❏ Pre-Weight-Bearing ❏ Tone Inhibition ■ Passive Trunk Elongation/Knee Hold ■ Passive Trunk Elongation/Pelvic Hold ■ Passive Trunk Elongation/Thoracic Hold ❏ Unilateral Upper Extremity ❏ Bilateral Upper Extremity ❏ Prone Unilateral Upper Extremity ❏ Unilateral Lower Extremity ■ Bilateral Lower Extremity ■ Bilateral Symmetrical Lower Extremity #1 ■ Bilateral Symmetrical Lower Extremity #2 ❏ Bilateral Reciprocal Lower Extremity ❏ Other: _____
Halliwick	❏ Phase I Adjustment ❏ Phase II Rotational Activities ❏ Turbulent Gliding ❏ Balance Training/Kangaroo Jumps ❏ Balance Training/Weight Shifting ❏ Other: _____

Cardiaquatics	❏ Level I Sequences: _____ Activities: ____
	❏ Level II Sequences: _____ Activities: ____
	❏ Level III Sequences: _____ Activities: ____
	❏ Level IV
	    ❏ Phase 1 ❏ Phase 2 ❏ Phase 3 ❏ All
	    ❏ Selected Sequences:

Other	■ Applied Myofascial Release ❏ Deep Friction Massage ❏ Applied Joint Mobilization/Distraction ■ Applied Spinal Mobilization/<u>Distraction</u> ❏ Applied Joint Approximation ❏ Applied Feldenkrais ❏ Applied Lymphatic Drainage ■ Watsu/Basic Flow ■ Watsu/Transitional Flow ■ Clinical Wassertanzen I ■ Clinical Wassertanzen II ■ Clinical Wassertanzen III ❏ Applied Aquatic Craniosacral Therapy ■ Trigger Point Therapy ■ Ai Chi: _____ ■ Spinal/Trunk Stabilization Protocol: ❏ Thoracic Outlet Syndrome Protocol: ❏ Other: _____

Functional / Goal Specific Aquatic Therapy Activities and Exercises

- ■ Gait Training (Forward/Backward) Laps: *1-5*
- ❏ Stair Climbing x _____
- ■ Bicycling Reps: _____
- ❏ Prone Activities Min _____
- ■ Aquajogging Laps: *2/min*
- ■ Heel Cord Stretch
- ■ Iliopsoas Stretch
- ■ Piriformis Stretch
- ■ TFL Stretch
- ■ IT Band Stretch
- ■ Hip Add Stretch
- ❏ Stork Stand
- ❏ Front to Back Weight Shifting
- ❏ Side to Side Weight Shifting
- ❏ Heel Raises Reps: _____
- ❏ Four-Corner Pivot Reps: _____

- ■ Side-Stepping Laps: _____
- ❏ Cross Over Stepping Laps: _____
- ❏ Deep-Water Stride Jump Reps: ____
- ■ Deep-Water Jogging (fwd/retro): *5* min.
- ❏ Deep-Water Groin Stretch
- ■ Knee to Chest Reps: _____
- ❏ Closed Kinematic Chain Exercises
- ■ Deep-Water Double Knee Lifts Reps: *20*
- ■ Wall Slide Reps: ____
- ■ Pelvic Tilts Reps: *20*
- ❏ Supine Kicks Reps:____
- ■ Deep-Water Spinal Traction in Vertical Suspension (*12* lbs. x *20* min.)
- ❏ Resistive Exercises:
- ❏ Other:_____

Aquatic Work Conditioning

- ❏ Resistive Forward/Retro Gait x _____ laps
- ❏ Deep-Water Jogging (fwd/retro) x _____ min.
- ❏ Tethered Jogging # ____ x _____ min.
- ❏ Swimming: _____laps/min

- ❏ Other:_____

Equipment Used

- ■ Bodyfit® Collar
- ❏ Floatation Vest
- ❏ Tire Tube
- ■ Floatation Pelvic Belt
- ❏ Fins
- ❏ Snorkel Mask
- ❏ Snorkel Tube
- ■ Ankle Floats
- ❏ Aqua-Dumbbells

- ■ AquaJogger
- ❏ Graduated-Resistance Paddles
- ❏ Hydrotone Boots
- ❏ Hoola Hoop
- ❏ Resistance Cord
- ❏ Thera-Band®
- ❏ Aquakinetic Machines
- ■ Boards
- ■ Floatation Noodle

- ❏ Hydrotone Dumbbells
- ❏ Weights: _____
- ■ Bad Ragaz Floatation Rings
- ■ Swim Bar
- ■ Recumbent Bicycle
- ❏ Underwater Treadmill
- ❏ Halliwick Blow Balls
- ❏ Other:_____

Adjunct Therapy

- ❏ Not Applicable

- ■ Whirlpool: *5-10* min. (spa)

- ■ Patient Education

- ■ Posture and Body Mechanics

- ■ Home Exercise Program

- ❏ Other:_____

Land Based Therapy Treatments

- ❏ Not Applicable

Frequency: _____ times per week
    for _____ weeks
- ■ US: *prn 1.5 w/cm²*
- ❏ ES: _____

- ❏ HP's: _____
- ■ Massage: *low back and gluteal region*
- ■ Piriformis Release *bilateral but emphasis on rt.*
- ❏ Therapeutic Exercises (specify):

- ❏ Paraffin Bath:

- ❏ Cryotherapy:

- ❏ Joint Mobilization:

- ❏ Other:

Comments:

_____   _____
Signature & Credentials of Therapist   Date

Discussion

The results of the manual muscle test seem to indicate that this patient has a right-sided disc herniation. However, in some muscle groups there is bilateral involvement. This is secondary to the high level of localized and radiated pain and it is also consistent with limitations of range of motion found and documented in the affected areas. Evidence of severe spasmodic activity of the external rotators suggests piriformis syndrome onset. The distribution of the pain in the right lower extremity and sensory impairment in the right calf confirms sciatic nerve compression secondary to piriformis tightness. Deviations in postural alignment as well as the antalgic gait are the result of the guarded posture that the patient assumes due to the high degree of pain. If the sciatic nerve is involved, the patient will present a positive Straight Leg Raise test and Fabere sign particularly in the side where the herniation has occurred. Vertebral glides at this level will additionally trigger the onset of pain.

There are a myriad of aquatic therapy interventions that may help achieve the established goals for the patient with low back pain. The key is to gradually integrate these interventions into the plan of care as symptoms diminish. The selected Bad Ragaz patterns promote movement, which decreases the pressure in the lumbar spine. Knee to chest movements or positions where the hip and knee are flexed provide an effective release of pressure on the spinal nerve root and decreasing radicular pain. Resistance may be applied as the pain decreases for strengthening purposes.

When soft tissue tightness occurs, the myofascial tissue also becomes affected limiting flexibility and movement further. Applied myofascial release techniques may be applied with the patient in the supine position wearing floatation devices. A very effective technique for releasing the myofascial tissue in aquatic rehabilitation is the application of the plunger technique. A small handheld plunger with a suction cup is used to release tight myofascia. For best results, the patient should either be sitting or in the cube position facing the wall with the therapist facing the patient's back. Furthermore, the Clinical Wassertanzen Protocol has maneuvers aimed at releasing the myofascial tissue. Distraction of the lumbar spine will further release nerve root compression. Integrated manual distraction in Watsu® or Clinical Wassertanzen may be applied to release nerve root compression. However, the most effective of all treatment techniques is vertical suspension in deep water using weights to enhance spinal distraction. Patients generally experience a significant decrease in localized and radiated pain. Trigger point releases are effective in decreasing localized muscle spasms and increased Ia and II fiber activity in the muscle. Using surface anatomy techniques, the therapist searches for the highest point of pain and spasmodic activity in the muscle, which is referred to as the trigger point. He then applies pressure until there is a release of the soft tissue and a decrease in pain.

Achieving optimal levels of relaxation and stress release through the application of Watsu® is necessary for the patient to experience a decrease in pain and for optimal results in the inhibition of soft tissue tightness. The second phase of the Clinical Wassertanzen Protocol integrate maneuvers and techniques that are directed at this objective. If the patient is proficient in the submersion phase, the outcomes might be even better. Therefore, it is advised to practice the three phases of breathing control if the Clinical Wassertanzen Protocol is considered.

Integrating an Ai Chi program into the plan of care might help to promote mobility and flexibility of the spine and pelvis in relation to the extremities. Additionally, the deep breathing activities that are associated with the Ai Chi Program work on further enhancing relaxation.

Shallow-water dynamic activities include stretching, selected gait activities, the use of the recumbent bicycle, and practice of adapted exercises for low-back pain. Deep-water dynamic activities are most effective in decreasing pain because of the lower impact on the spine and extremities. Forward deep-water jogging with retroactivity is just as effective as the vertical suspen-

sion technique for spinal distraction using weights. It is vital to monitor pain levels in these patients prior to and after the aquatic therapy session. If the patient reports extremely high pain levels prior to the session, rendering him unable to perform the selected activities, the session should begin with twenty minutes of vertical suspension followed by a number of deep-water jogging laps.

Supplementary interventions are necessary depending on the degree of involvement. In this case, the patient's primary problem has been compounded by the onset of piriformis syndrome and related signs. Therefore, integrating land-based approaches might complement the plan of care and facilitate the expected outcomes. Manual piriformis release should be considered with possible additional ultrasound applications and therapeutic massage.

APPENDICES

The DASI forms referenced in the text are shown on the following pages:

DASI
Diagnostic Aquatics-Systems Integration — Pre-Aquatic Therapy Assessment

Patient Name: _____ Date: _____

Dx: _____ Age: _____

History/Problems/Complaints:

Clinical Impression:

Musculoskeletal Assessment

Musculoskeletal Assessment		Manual Muscle Test		Range of Motion	
		Right	Left	Right	Left
Shoulder	Flexors				
	Extensors				
	Abductors				
	Adductors				
	External Rotators				
	Internal Rotators				
Elbow	Flexors				
	Extensors				
Forearm	Pronators				
	Supinators				
Wrist	Flexors				
	Extensors				
Finger	Flexors/Hand Grip				
Hip	Flexors				
	Extensors				
	Abductors				
	Adductors				
	External Rotators				
	Internal Rotators				

Musculoskeletal Assessment		Manual Muscle Test		Range of Motion	
		Right	Left	Right	Left
Knee	Flexors				
	Extensors				
Ankle	Dorsiflexors				
	Plantar Flexors				
Foot	Invertors				
	Evertors				

Musculoskeletal Assessment	MMT	ROM
Cervical Flexion		
Cervical Extension		
Cervical Lateral Flexion (right)		
Cervical Lateral Flexion (left)		
Cervical Rotation (right)		
Cervical Rotation (left)		
Lumbar Flexion		
Lumbar Extension		
Lumbar Lateral Flexion (right)		
Lumbar Lateral Flexion (left)		

(Spine)

Evidence of Edema? ❏ Yes ❏ No

Girth Anatomical Landmark: ____ ❏Not Applicable

Right:	_____inch(es)	Left:	_____ inch(es)

Leg-Length Discrepancy? ❏ Yes ❏ No
Approximate Discrepancy: _____ inch(es)

Musculoskeletal Assessment (continued)

Posture	
Posture	**Posture**
	❏ Normal Alignment
	❏ Postural Deviations
	Explain

Spasmodic Activity					
❏ No evidence of muscle spasms	**Grade**				
❏ Not applicable	**1**	**2**	**3**	**4**	

Spasmodic Activity	**Muscles**				

Cardiopulmonary Assessment

Lungs

❏ Clear to Auscultation
❏ Abnormal Breath Sounds

❏ Adventitious Breath Sounds

❏ Resonant Chest to Mediate Percussion
❏ Other:

❏ Bibasilar Thoracic Asymmetry

RR: _____ ❏ Normal ❏ Dyspnea ❏ Other:

Cardiac

	Other:
❏ Normal S1	
❏ Normal S2	
❏ Split S1	
❏ Split S2	
❏ S3	
❏ S4	
❏ Murmur	
❏ Ejection Click	
HR: _____	
BP: _____	

Neurological Assessment

Neurologic Assessment	
Superficial Sensation	❏ Intact **Explain** ❏ Impaired
Coordination	❏ Intact **Explain** ❏ Impaired ❏ Intention Tremors
Proprioception	❏ Intact **Explain** ❏ Impaired
Deep Tendon Reflexes	❏ Intact **Explain** ❏ Diminished _____ ❏ Hyperactive _____
Balance	Static ❏ Intact ❏ Impaired Dynamic ❏ Intact ❏ Impaired

Pain

No Pain   Intolerable Pain
0   1   2   3   4   5   6   7   8   9   10

Tone

❏ Normal
❏ Hypertonia / Spasticity

❏ Hypotonia / Flaccidity

❏ Cogwheel Rigidity

❏ Contractures

Other Neurologic Test Results

	Check the Appropriate Box		
	Pos	**Neg**	**N/A**
SLR Test	❏	❏	❏
Neural Tension	❏	❏	❏
___ Ulnar ___ Radial ___ Median			
Fabere Sign	❏	❏	❏
Compression Test	❏	❏	❏
Distraction Stretch	❏	❏	❏
Vertebral Artery Test	❏	❏	❏
Alar Ligament Test	❏	❏	❏
Vertebral Glide Test	❏	❏	❏
Babinski Sign	❏	❏	❏
Romberg's Test	❏	❏	❏
Other	❏	❏	❏

Functional Assessment

Mobility		
Gait Analysis	❏ Ambulatory ❏Non-Ambulatory Explain: ❏ Assistive Device: Weight Bearing: ❏ FWB ❏ PWB ❏ NWB ❏ No significant gait deviations noted. ❏ Gait Deviations: ❏ Abnormal Gait:	
Bed Mobility	❏ Independent ❏ Requires assistance ❏ max ❏ mod ❏ min	
Transfers	❏ Independent ❏ Requires assistance ❏ max ❏ mod ❏ min	
Body Mechanics	❏ Not tested ❏ Uses proper body mechanics when lifting, carrying, sitting, and lying down ❏ Does not use proper body mechanics when lifting, carrying, and lying down ❏ Needs further instruction and practice	

Goals

❏ Improve endurance
❏ Improve balance
❏ Improve spinal mobility
❏ Promote relaxation
❏ Improve breathing patterns

❏ Decrease pain

❏ Increase muscle strength

❏ Increase joint range and flexibility

❏ Improve gait pattern
❏ Improve coordination and proprioception
❏ Reduce muscle fatigue
❏ Decrease edema and inflammation

❏ Improve postural alignment
❏ Improve circulation
❏ Improve motor control
❏ Inhibit spasticity/hypertonicity

❏ Resolution of muscle spasms:

Plan of Care

Frequency: ____ times per week for ____ weeks

Bad Ragaz	❏ Passive Relaxation ❏ Passive Pelvic Tilts ❏ Pre-Gait ❏ Isotonic #1 ❏ Isotonic #2 ❏ Isometric ❏ Pre-Weight-Bearing ❏ Tone Inhibition ❏ Passive Trunk Elongation/Knee Hold ❏ Passive Trunk Elongation/Pelvic Hold ❏ Passive Trunk Elongation/Thoracic Hold ❏ Unilateral Upper Extremity ❏ Bilateral Upper Extremity ❏ Prone Unilateral Upper Extremity ❏ Unilateral Lower Extremity ❏ Bilateral Lower Extremity ❏ Bilateral Symmetrical Lower Extremity #1 ❏ Bilateral Symmetrical Lower Extremity #2 ❏ Bilateral Reciprocal Lower Extremity ❏ Other: _____
Halliwick	❏ Phase I Adjustment ❏ Phase II Rotational Activities ❏ Turbulent Gliding ❏ Balance Training/Kangaroo Jumps ❏ Balance Training/Weight Shifting ❏ Other: _____

Cardiaquatics	❏ Level I Sequences: _____ Activities: ____
	❏ Level II Sequences: _____ Activities: ____
	❏ Level III Sequences: _____ Activities: ____
	❏ Level IV
	   ❏ Phase 1 ❏ Phase 2 ❏ Phase 3 ❏ All
	   ❏ Selected Sequences:

Other	❏ Applied Myofascial Release ❏ Deep Friction Massage ❏ Applied Joint Mobilization/Distraction ❏ Applied Spinal Mobilization/Distraction ❏ Applied Joint Approximation ❏ Applied Feldenkrais ❏ Applied Lymphatic Drainage ❏ Watsu/Basic Flow ❏ Watsu/Transitional Flow ❏ Clinical Wassertanzen I ❏ Clinical Wassertanzen II ❏ Clinical Wassertanzen III ❏ Applied Aquatic Craniosacral Therapy ❏ Trigger Point Therapy ❏ Ai Chi: _____ ❏ Spinal/Trunk Stabilization Protocol: ❏ Thoracic Outlet Syndrome Protocol: ❏ Other: _____

Functional / Goal Specific Aquatic Therapy Activities and Exercises

❐ Gait Training (Forward/Backward) Laps: _____
❐ Stair Climbing x _____
❐ Bicycling Reps: _____
❐ Prone Activities Min _____
❐ Aquajogging Laps: _____
❐ Heel Cord Stretch
❐ Iliopsoas Stretch
❐ Piriformis Stretch
❐ TFL Stretch
❐ IT Band Stretch
❐ Hip Add Stretch
❐ Stork Stand
❐ Front to Back Weight Shifting
❐ Side to Side Weight Shifting
❐ Heel Raises Reps: _____
❐ Four-Corner Pivot Reps: _____

❐ Side Stepping Laps: _____
❐ Cross Over Stepping Laps: _____
❐ Deep-Water Stride Jump Reps: _____
❐ Deep-Water Jogging (fwd/retro): _____ min.
❐ Deep-Water Groin Stretch
❐ Knee to Chest Reps: _____
❐ Closed Kinematic Chain Exercises
❐ Deep-Water Double Knee Lifts Reps: _____
❐ Wall Slide Reps: _____
❐ Pelvic Tilts Reps: _____
❐ Supine Kicks Reps: _____
❐ Deep-Water Spinal Traction in Vertical Suspension
    (_____ lbs. x _____ min.)
❐ Resistive Exercises:

❐ Other:_____

Aquatic Work Conditioning

❐ Resistive Forward/Retro Gait x _____ laps
❐ Deep-Water Jogging (fwd/retro) x _____ min.
❐ Tethered Jogging # _____ x _____ min.

❐ Swimming: _____laps/min
❐ Other:_____

Equipment Used

❐ Bodyfit® Collar
❐ Floatation Vest
❐ Tire Tube
❐ Floatation Pelvic Belt
❐ Fins
❐ Snorkel Mask
❐ Snorkel Tube
❐ Ankle Floats
❐ Aqua-Dumbbells

❐ AquaJogger
❐ Graduated-Resistance Paddles
❐ Hydrotone Boots
❐ Hoola Hoop
❐ Resistance Cord
❐ Thera-Band®
❐ Aquakinetic Machines
❐ Boards
❐ Floatation Noodle

❐ Hydrotone Dumbbells
❐ Weights: _____
❐ Bad Ragaz Floatation Rings
❐ Swim Bar
❐ Recumbent Bicycle
❐ Underwater Treadmill
❐ Halliwick Blow Balls
❐ Other:_____

Adjunct Therapy

❐ Not Applicable

❐ Whirlpool: _____ min. (spa)

❐ Patient Education

❐ Posture and Body Mechanics

❐ Home Exercise Program

❐ Other:_____

Land Based Therapy Treatments

❐ Not Applicable

Frequency: _____ times per week
        for _____ weeks
❐ US: _____
❐ ES: _____

❐ HP's: _____
❐ Massage: _____
❐ Piriformis Release
❐ Therapeutic Exercises (specify):

❐ Paraffin Bath:

❐ Cryotherapy:

❐ Joint Mobilization:

❐ Other:

Comments:

_____   _____
Signature & Credentials of Therapist   Date

DASI — Post-Therapy
Diagnostic Aquatics-Systems Integration — Post-Aquatic Therapy Reassessment

Patient Name: _____ Date: _____

Dx: _____ Age: _____

History/Problems/Complaints:

Clinical Impression:

Musculoskeletal Assessment

Musculoskeletal Assessment		Manual Muscle Test		Range of Motion	
		Right	Left	Right	Left
Shoulder	Flexors				
	Extensors				
	Abductors				
	Adductors				
	External Rotators				
	Internal Rotators				
Elbow	Flexors				
	Extensors				
Forearm	Pronators				
	Supinators				
Wrist	Flexors				
	Extensors				
Finger	Flexors/Hand Grip				
Hip	Flexors				
	Extensors				
	Abductors				
	Adductors				
	External Rotators				
	Internal Rotators				

Musculoskeletal Assessment		Manual Muscle Test		Range of Motion	
		Right	Left	Right	Left
Knee	Flexors				
	Extensors				
Ankle	Dorsiflexors				
	Plantar Flexors				
Foot	Invertors				
	Evertors				

Musculoskeletal Assessment	MMT	ROM
Cervical Flexion		
Cervical Extension		
Cervical Lateral Flexion (right)		
Cervical Lateral Flexion (left)		
Cervical Rotation (right)		
Cervical Rotation (left)		
Lumbar Flexion		
Lumbar Extension		
Lumbar Lateral Flexion (right)		
Lumbar Lateral Flexion (left)		

(Spine applies to the Cervical and Lumbar rows above)

Evidence of Edema?   ❏ Yes   ❏ No

Girth Anatomical Landmark: _____ ❏Not Applicable		
Right:	_____ inch(es)	Left:	_____ inch(es)

Leg-Length Discrepancy?   ❏ Yes   ❏ No
Approximate Discrepancy: _____ inch(es)

Musculoskeletal Assessment (continued)

Posture

	Posture
Posture	❏ Normal Alignment ❏ Postural Deviations Explain

Spasmodic Activity

		Grade			
	❏ No evidence of muscle spasms ❏ Not applicable	**1**	**2**	**3**	**4**
Spasmodic Activity	**Muscles**				

Cardiopulmonary Assessment

Lungs	❏ Clear to Auscultation ❏ Abnormal Breath Sounds ❏ Adventitious Breath Sounds ❏ Resonant Chest to Mediate Percussion ❏ Other: ❏ Bibasilar Thoracic Asymmetry RR: _____ ❏ Normal ❏ Dyspnea ❏ Other:	
Cardiac	❏ Normal S1 ❏ Normal S2 ❏ Split S1 ❏ Split S2 ❏ S3 ❏ S4 ❏ Murmur ❏ Ejection Click HR: _____ BP: _____	Other:

Neurological Assessment

Neurologic Assessment

Superficial Sensation	❏ Intact ❏ Impaired	**Explain**
Coordination	❏ Intact ❏ Impaired ❏ Intention Tremors	**Explain**
Proprioception	❏ Intact ❏ Impaired	**Explain**
Deep Tendon Reflexes	❏ Intact ❏ Diminished _____ ❏ Hyperactive _____	**Explain**
Balance	Static ❏ Intact ❏ Impaired Dynamic ❏ Intact ❏ Impaired	

Pain	No Pain Intolerable Pain 0 1 2 3 4 5 6 7 8 9 10
Tone	❏ Normal ❏ Hypertonia / Spasticity ❏ Hypotonia / Flaccidity ❏ Cogwheel Rigidity ❏ Contractures

		Check the Appropriate Box		
		Pos	**Neg**	**N/A**
Other Neurologic Test Results	SLR Test	❏	❏	❏
	Neural Tension	❏	❏	❏
	Ulnar Radial Median			
	Fabere Sign	❏	❏	❏
	Compression Test	❏	❏	❏
	Distraction Stretch	❏	❏	❏
	Vertebral Artery Test	❏	❏	❏
	Alar Ligament Test	❏	❏	❏
	Vertebral Glide Test	❏	❏	❏
	Babinski Sign	❏	❏	❏
	Romberg's Test	❏	❏	❏
	Other	❏	❏	❏

Functional Assessment

	Mobility	
Gait Analysis	❏ Ambulatory ❏ Non-Ambulatory Explain: ❏ Assistive Device: Weight Bearing: ❏ FWB ❏ PWB ❏ NWB ❏ No significant gait deviations noted. ❏ Gait Deviations: ❏ Abnormal Gait:	
Bed Mobility	❏ Independent ❏ Requires assistance ❏ max ❏ mod ❏ min	
Transfers	❏ Independent ❏ Requires assistance ❏ max ❏ mod ❏ min	
Body Mechanics	❏ Not tested ❏ Uses proper body mechanics when lifting, carrying, sitting, and lying down ❏ Does not use proper body mechanics when lifting, carrying, and lying down ❏ Needs further instruction and practice	

Goal Attainment

(Check goals in plan and level attained.)

❏ Improve endurance ❏25 ❏50 ❏75 ❏100%
❏ Improve balance ❏25 ❏50 ❏75 ❏100%
❏ Improve spinal mobility ❏25 ❏50 ❏75 ❏100%
❏ Promote relaxation ❏25 ❏50 ❏75 ❏100%
❏ Improve breathing patterns
 ❏25 ❏50 ❏75 ❏100%
❏ Decrease pain ❏25 ❏50 ❏75 ❏100%
❏ Increase muscle strength ❏25 ❏50 ❏75 ❏100%
❏ Increase joint range and flexibility
 ❏25 ❏50 ❏75 ❏100%
❏ Improve gait pattern ❏25 ❏50 ❏75 ❏100%
❏ Improve coordination and proprioception
 ❏25 ❏50 ❏75 ❏100%
❏ Reduce muscle fatigue ❏25 ❏50 ❏75 ❏100%
❏ Decrease edema and inflammation
 ❏25 ❏50 ❏75 ❏100%
❏ Improve postural alignment
 ❏25 ❏50 ❏75 ❏100%
❏ Improve circulation ❏25 ❏50 ❏75 ❏100%
❏ Improve motor control ❏25 ❏50 ❏75 ❏100%
❏ Inhibit spasticity/hypertonicity
 ❏25 ❏50 ❏75 ❏100%
❏ Resolution of muscle spasms:
 ❏25 ❏50 ❏75 ❏100%

Plan of Care Summary

Frequency: ____ times per week for ____ weeks

Bad Ragaz	❏ Passive Relaxation ❏ Passive Pelvic Tilts ❏ Pre-Gait ❏ Isotonic #1 ❏ Isotonic #2 ❏ Isometric ❏ Pre-Weight-Bearing ❏ Tone Inhibition ❏ Passive Trunk Elongation/Knee Hold ❏ Passive Trunk Elongation/Pelvic Hold ❏ Passive Trunk Elongation/Thoracic Hold ❏ Unilateral Upper Extremity ❏ Bilateral Upper Extremity ❏ Prone Unilateral Upper Extremity ❏ Unilateral Lower Extremity ❏ Bilateral Lower Extremity ❏ Bilateral Symmetrical Lower Extremity #1 ❏ Bilateral Symmetrical Lower Extremity #2 ❏ Bilateral Reciprocal Lower Extremity ❏ Other: _____
Halliwick	❏ Phase I Adjustment ❏ Phase II Rotational Activities ❏ Turbulent Gliding ❏ Balance Training/Kangaroo Jumps ❏ Balance Training/Weight Shifting ❏ Other: _____

Cardiaquatics	❏ Level I Sequences: _____ Activities: ____
	❏ Level II Sequences: _____ Activities: ____
	❏ Level III Sequences: _____ Activities: ____
	❏ Level IV
	   ❏ Phase 1 ❏ Phase 2 ❏ Phase 3 ❏ All
	      ❏ Selected Sequences:

Other	❏ Applied Myofascial Release ❏ Deep Friction Massage ❏ Applied Joint Mobilization/Distraction ❏ Applied Spinal Mobilization/Distraction ❏ Applied Joint Approximation ❏ Applied Feldenkrais ❏ Applied Lymphatic Drainage ❏ Watsu/Basic Flow ❏ Watsu/Transitional Flow ❏ Clinical Wassertanzen I ❏ Clinical Wassertanzen II ❏ Clinical Wassertanzen III ❏ Applied Aquatic Craniosacral Therapy ❏ Trigger Point Therapy ❏ Ai Chi: _____ ❏ Spinal/Trunk Stabilization Protocol: _____ ❏ Thoracic Outlet Syndrome Protocol: _____ ❏ Other: _____

Functional / Goal Specific Aquatic Therapy Activities and Exercises

❏ Gait Training (Forward/Backward) Laps: _____
❏ Stair Climbing x _____
❏ Bicycling Reps: _____
❏ Prone Activities Min: _____
❏ Aquajogging Laps: _____
❏ Heel Cord Stretch
❏ Iliopsoas Stretch
❏ Piriformis Stretch
❏ TFL Stretch
❏ IT Band Stretch
❏ Hip Add Stretch
❏ Stork Stand
❏ Front to Back Weight Shifting
❏ Side to Side Weight Shifting
❏ Heel Raises Reps: _____
❏ Four-Corner Pivot Reps: _____

❏ Side Stepping Laps: _____
❏ Cross Over Stepping Laps: _____
❏ Deep-Water Stride Jump Reps: _____
❏ Deep-Water Jogging (fwd/retro): _____ min.
❏ Deep-Water Groin Stretch
❏ Knee to Chest Reps: _____
❏ Closed Kinematic Chain Exercises
❏ Deep-Water Double Knee Lifts Reps: _____
❏ Wall Slide Reps: _____
❏ Pelvic Tilts Reps: _____
❏ Supine Kicks Reps:_____
❏ Deep-Water Spinal Traction in Vertical Suspension
   (_____ lbs. x _____ min.)
❏ Resistive Exercises:

❏ Other:_____

Aquatic Work Conditioning

❏ Resistive Forward/Retro Gait x _____ laps
❏ Deep-Water Jogging (fwd/retro) x _____ min.
❏ Tethered Jogging # _____ x _____ min.

❏ Swimming: _____laps/min
❏ Other:_____

Equipment Used

❏ Bodyfit® Collar
❏ Floatation Vest
❏ Tire Tube
❏ Floatation Pelvic Belt
❏ Fins
❏ Snorkel Mask
❏ Snorkel Tube
❏ Ankle Floats
❏ Aqua-Dumbbells

❏ AquaJogger
❏ Graduated-Resistance Paddles
❏ Hydrotone Boots
❏ Hoola Hoop
❏ Resistance Cord
❏ Thera-Band®
❏ Aquakinetic Machines
❏ Boards
❏ Floatation Noodle

❏ Hydrotone Dumbbells
❏ Weights: _____
❏ Bad Ragaz Floatation Rings
❏ Swim Bar
❏ Recumbent Bicycle
❏ Underwater Treadmill
❏ Halliwick Blow Balls
❏ Other:_____

Adjunct Therapy

❏ Not Applicable

❏ Whirlpool: _____ min. (spa)

❏ Patient Education

❏ Posture and Body Mechanics

❏ Home Exercise Program

❏ Other:_____

Land Based Therapy Treatments

❏ Not Applicable

Frequency: _____ times per week
         for _____ weeks
❏ US: _____
❏ ES: _____

❏ HP's: _____
❏ Massage: _____
❏ Piriformis Release
❏ Therapeutic Exercises (specify):

❏ Paraffin Bath:

❏ Cryotherapy:

❏ Joint Mobilization:

❏ Other:

Recommendation

❏ Discharge patient from Aquatic Physical Therapy due
   to goal attainment
❏ Discharge patient from Aquatic Physical Therapy due
   to goal noncompliance
❏ Patient has not attained goals and requires further
   aquatic therapy sessions

❏ Discharge patient from Aquatic Physical Therapy due
   to noncompliance with appointments
❏ Renewal of Aquatic Physical Therapy Referral
❏ Extension of Aquatic Physical Therapy Referral for
   ____ additional treatments
❏ Modification of Aquatic Physical Therapy:
   _____

Comments:

_____   _____
Signature & Credentials of Therapist   Date

AQUATIC THERAPY PROGRESS NOTE

Date: _____
Subjective: Pre-Aquatic Therapy Pain Level _____ Location: _____
Additional Info: _____
_____

Objective: ☐ Shallow Water Dynamic Activities* ☐ Deep Water Dynamic Activities*
☐ Kinetic Activities*
☐ Specialized Interventions: ___ Bad Ragaz ___ Halliwick ___ Watsu
Other: _____
_____
☐ Pre-Aquatic Assessment ☐ Post-Aquatic Assessment Therapist's Initials: _____
☐ Land-based Techniques: _____

Assessment: ☐ Status quo ☐ Condition improved ☐ Condition Worsened
☐ Progressing towards goal attainment* ☐ Responding/Tolerated Rx well
☐ Motivated/Cooperative ☐ Unmotivated/Uncooperative
Post Aquatic Therapy Pain Level ___ Location: _____
Clinical Observations: _____
_____
_____

Plan: ☐ Continue as outlined on DASI Pre-Aquatic Assessment. Follow established Plan of Care.
☐ Integrate the following Modifications or Recommendations: _____
_____
_____Therapist only/Initials: _____
* **Refer to DASI Pre-Aquatic Assessment**
Signature and Credentials: _____

Date: _____
Subjective: Pre-Aquatic Therapy Pain Level _____ Location: _____
Additional Info: _____
_____

Objective: ☐ Shallow Water Dynamic Activities* ☐ Deep Water Dynamic Activities*
☐ Kinetic Activities*
☐ Specialized Interventions: ___ Bad Ragaz ___ Halliwick ___ Watsu
Other: _____
_____
☐ Pre-Aquatic Assessment ☐ Post-Aquatic Assessment Therapist's Initials: _____
☐ Land-based Techniques: _____

Assessment: ☐ Status quo ☐ Condition improved ☐ Condition Worsened
☐ Progressing towards goal attainment* ☐ Responding/Tolerated Rx well
☐ Motivated/Cooperative ☐ Unmotivated/Uncooperative
Post Aquatic Therapy Pain Level ___ Location: _____
Clinical Observations: _____
_____
_____

Plan: ☐ Continue as outlined on DASI Pre-Aquatic Assessment. Follow established Plan of Care.
☐ Integrate the following Modifications or Recommendations: _____
_____
_____Therapist only/Initials: _____
* **Refer to DASI Pre-Aquatic Assessment**
Signature and Credentials: _____

Patient's Name: _____

Dx: _____

Cardiaquatics Flow Sheet

Preactivity Heart Rate: _____   **Preactivity Blood Pressure:** _____

Date	Level	Sequence	Activity	HR	Comments, Blood Pressure, or Pulmonary Function Reading

Pre-Wata* Pulmonary Function Readings: _____Insp. Cap. _____% SaO_2 _____VC
Post-Wata* Pulmonary Function Readings: _____Insp. Cap. _____% SaO_2 _____VC

*Wata = Wassertanzen

GLOSSARY

abdominals the muscles that form the anterior and lateral wall of the abdomen. These are the rectus abdominis, the external oblique and internal oblique, and the transversus abdominis.

ABG abbreviation for arterial blood gases.

acetabulum the cup-like depression located on the lateral aspect of the junction of the three bones that form the hip joint. The head of the femur articulates directly with the acetabulum to form the hip joint. The plural of acetabulum is acetabula.

acromioclavicular joint the joint formed by the union of the acromion process (a flat bony landmark) formed by the scapula and the lateral end of the clavicle. Also called the scapuloclavicular joint.

acromioclavicular ligaments the fibrous bands that bind the acromioclavicular joint on all aspects and provide stability to the clavicle/scapula joint.

adductor brevis a short muscle that facilitates movement of the thigh toward midline; part of the *adductors of the hip*.

adductor magnus the great or largest adductor of the thigh; one of the *adductors of the hip*.

adductors of the hip the adductors of the hip (or thigh) consist of six muscles that move the femur towards the mid-line. These are the adductor magnus, adductor longus, adductor brevis, gracilis, pectineus, and adductor minimus.

afferent literally meaning to bring toward the center. Specific to neurology, a pathway that begins at a receptor where the stimulus is received and carries the stimulus to the central nervous system where it is interpreted. Opposite of *efferent*.

agonist 1. [physiology] the primary anatomical structure or muscle responsible for a movement. 2. [pharmacology] a drug that stimulates activity or movement at cell receptors that are normally stimulated by naturally occurring substances in the body.

alar ligament the ligament that binds the dens or odontoid process of the axis (second cervical vertebra) to the foramen magnum, the large opening at the base of the skull that allows passage of the spinal cord. The ligament emerges from each side of the dens forming two wings ("alar" means winglike) and attaches to the border of the foramen magnum.

amphi- implying double, or corresponding to both sides.

amphiarthrodial joint two joint surfaces joined together by cartilage and supported by ligaments. Amphiarthrodial joints allow only moderate movement (range of motion), which is achieved through the flexing of either ligaments or cartilage. There are two different types of amphiarthrodial joints: syndesmosis (joints bound together by ligaments such as the tibiofibular joint) and synchondrosis (joints bound together by cartilage such as the costochondral joints that join the ribs to the sternum). Another example of an amphiarthrodial joint is the sacroiliac joint where the irregular articular surfaces of the sacrum articulate with the irregular surfaces of the ilium.

ankle joint　the joint formed by the union of the leg bones, tibia and fibula, and the talus. These form the mortise and allow dorsiflexion (where the foot moves up towards the leg) and plantar flexion (where the foot moves down away from the leg). See also *subtaler joint.*

anterolateral　anything that encompasses or covers two areas: 1. the anterior area or front of a surface and 2. the lateral area or outside of a surface. An example would be the cheek area of the face, which is both anterior and lateral in the facial structure.

anteromedial　encompassing or covering two areas: 1. the anterior area or front of a surface and 2. the medial area or inside of a surface. For example, the eyes are normally on the front of the face toward the middle, near the nose.

anteroposterior　anything that encompasses or covers two areas: 1. the anterior area or front of a surface and 2. the posterior area or back of a surface.

anteroposterior axis　an imaginary vector that is aimed in a direction from the front of a segment, through the segment, and exiting the back of the segment that it crosses.

apneustic center　a specialized respiratory sub-center located in the reticular formation of the medulla oblongata and pons, which is only activated when the activity of the respiratory pacemaker, the pneumotaxic center, slows down.

appendicular　the appendages, limbs, or extremities; that is, the two upper extremities and the two lower extremities. The anatomical counterpart to *axial*, which refers to the head and trunk.

Aquacalisthenics　warm-up exercises performed in the water with the objectives of achieving respiratory and musculoskeletal adjustments and preparing the cardiovascular system for more vigorous exercises. Developed by Dr. Luis G. Vargas.

aquakinetics　the study of the physical and biological processes involved in moving through water including resistance, force, and rate.

arterial blood gases　the primary arterial gases are oxygen (P_aO_2 – sometimes written as pO_2) and carbon dioxide (P_aCO_2 – sometimes written as pCO_2). These represent the arterial pressure at which oxygen and carbon dioxide diffuse in plasma through the alveolar-capillary membrane. Bicarbonate (HCO_3), which is manufactured in the kidneys, is also considered an important blood gas value that regulates the internal process of respiration in the lungs. Along with the pH of the arterial blood, these arterial blood gases help the therapist determine if the problem is respiratory or metabolic and provide evidence of acidemia or alkalemia.

arthrokinematics　the science that studies the relationship between joint surfaces and how they produce movement. This is different than *osteokinematics*, which refers to the study of joint movement.

arthroplasty   surgical repair or replacement of a joint.

articular referring to a joint; allowing movement.

articulate 1. made up of multiple bones forming a joint that allows motion, often referred to as articulation instead of articulate. 2. ability to distinctly pronounce words by manipulating one's vocal organs and body structure.

atelectasis   the partial or complete collapse of a lung segment or lobe due to inadequate ventilation. It can occur from an obstructed airway, fibrosis as part of a disease process, or from pressure created in the chest cavity.

atlantoaxial joint the joint or articulation between the atlas (first cervical vertebra) and axis (second cervical vertebra).

atlanto-occipital joint   the joint or articulation between the atlas (first cervical vertebra) and the condyles of the occipital bone (the bone at the base of the skull).

auscultate the examination procedure that involves listening to sounds inside of the body as a means to evaluate health status. Auscultation may or may not require the use of a stethoscope, depending on the protocol for the specific examination. Most commonly, auscultation of the heart and lungs requires the use of a stethoscope.

axial referring to the head and trunk.

Babinski sign a means to assess the presence of central nervous system damage (particularly a lesion in the pyramidal tract) in adult patients. The therapist runs his thumbnail or the pointed end of the reflex hammer from the patient's heal toward the big toe. If the patient's toes hyperextend (fan out)

and the big toe dorsiflexes up, the patient is considered to have a positive Babinski sign (positive for central nervous system damage). This "positive" Babinski sign applies to children and adults. In newborns a positive Babinski sign is normal.

biaxial joint a joint that moves around two axes.

biceps brachii named for its two heads of origin, this is the most superficial muscle of the anterior compartment of the arm responsible for flexing the elbow with supination but also functioning in flexion of the shoulder because it crosses that joint anteriorly.

biceps femoris   named for its two heads of origin, one of three muscles collectively known as the hamstrings, which acts as the primary flexor of the knee. The biceps femoris muscle is the most lateral of the hamstring muscles. Because the origin crosses the posterior axis of the hip joint, it also acts as an extensor of the hip joint if the action in the knee joint is isolated.

bicondylar joint a joint characterized by two condyles or rounded prominences articulating with a slight depression in the opposite surface.

Bodyfit® collar a trademarked floatation cervical collar used for several aquatic therapy interventions requiring floatation of the upper quarter of the body.

bronchospasm a constriction or narrowing of the airway, limiting the amount of oxygen inhaled and preventing carbon dioxide from being exhaled into the atmosphere. It is characterized by shortness of breath.

bronchovesicular sounds a type of normal breath sound, characterized by inspiratory and expiratory phases of equal length. Bronchovesicular sounds have soft, tubular quality. In the anterior check they are heard in the center; in the posterior check they are heard between the scapulae.

calcaneocuboid joint the joint between the heel bone (calcaneus) and the most lateral of the tarsals (the cuboid bone).

cannula a catheter-like device partially or fully inserted in the body. A nasal cannula is partially or fully inserted into the nostrils either to deliver oxygen via an oxygen source or to suction secretions from the airway if it is connected to a suction device.

cardiomyopathy a progressive disease or deterioration of the heart muscle or myocardium.

cardiorespiratory referring to the heart and lungs.

carpal joints the joint between the carpal bones in the hand. There are two rows of small bones called carpals. The proximal row, closest to the forearm, consists of the scaphoid, lunate, triquetrum, and pisiform. The distal row, closest to the metacarpals in the hand consists of the trapezium, trapezoid, capitate, and hammate.

carpometacarpal joint the joint between the distal row of carpal bones and the bases of the metacarpals of the hand, including the thumb.

cephalocaudal following a direction from the head to the feet or from the center of the body towards each end (the head and the feet).

cervico- pertaining to the cervical spine, or neck.

cervico-thoraco-lumbar involving the cervical, thoracic, and lumbar components of the spine.

Charcot's joint also known as a naturopathic joint. This is a pathological arthropathy characterized by a swollen, hypermobile but painless metatarsophalangeal joint with associated atrophy in the surrounding musculature. A Charcot's joint has diminished proprioceptive sensation and is often associated with neuropathy due to diabetes or the progressive wasting of tabes dorsalis.

chondrosternal joint the cartilage that joins the ribs to the sternum.

circumduction a circular movement that involves a combination of flexion, extension, abduction, adduction, internal rotation, and external rotation.

clinicopathologic referring to both the disease process and the symptoms associated with the disease process.

condylar joint a joint characterized by a convex rounded prominence known as a condyle articulating with a convex depression.

contralateral pertaining to the opposite side.

coracobrachialis a small muscle located near the axilla. This muscle attaches to the coracoid process of the scapula and the arm, and acts as a flexor of the shoulder.

coracoclavicular ligament the ligament that attaches to the coracoid process of the scapula and the clavicle providing support to these two bones and to the shoulder region.

costochondral joints the joints connecting the bony surface of the ribs with the rib cartilage.

costolateral breathing the movement of the rib cage in an outward direction to each side upon inhalation. The chest expands sideways and the ribs move laterally and upwards towards each other. This type of rib cage breathing involves activity of the intercostal muscles.

costotransverse joints the joints between the transverse processes of the thoracic vertebrae and the tubercles of the rib.

cryotherapy the use of cold for therapeutic purposes in the treatment of musculoskeletal, neurological, and integumentary conditions.

cubital the anatomical area covering the anterior aspect of the elbow joint marked by a crease or depression in the flexor region of the elbow joint.

CXR an abbreviation that stands for chest x- ray.

debridement the removal of necrotic or eschar tissue or foreign material from an injured area down to the level of healthy tissue.

decussation nerve fibers in the central nervous system crossing in the pattern of an X; results in the left brain controlling the right side of the body and vice versa.

deltoid the muscle that forms the contour of the shoulder and shapes the shoulder. It originates from the scapula and clavicle, attaches to the humerus. Although the entire muscle acts as an abductor of the shoulder, it is divided into three portions each of which have a specific function.

discectomy the surgical removal of an intervertebral disc following herniation of a disc that puts pressure on the nerve root. Also spelled "diskectomy."

dorsiflexion movement of the ankle where the foot moves upward toward the leg.

dyspnea difficulty with breathing.

ecchymosis patchy blue or purplish spots in the skin or membrane due to rupturing of blood vessels causing discoloration but not an elevated level of the skin or membrane.

effector organ an organ that causes a response in the body such as dorsiflexion of the foot or secreting endorphins in response to a scare. Muscles are effector organs. For muscles, this term refers to the site where the response from the stimulus occurs once it is received by the afferent pathway into the central nervous system, interpreted and sent through the efferent pathway to the organ that will display the response.

efferent literally to move outward. Neurologically, a nerve impulse from a nerve center (e.g., brain or spinal cord) to cause some type of action such as a muscle contraction, release of a glandular secretion, or discharge a small electrical current. See *afferent.*

erector spinae the primary muscle that extends the spine. It consists of three components: the iliocostalis, the longissimus, and the spinalis. The muscle and its components cover all the various sections of the spine and, depending on their location, they are termed cervicis, thoracis, or lumborum.

erythema redness in the skin surface that might indicate inflammation and be associated with swelling and tenderness.

eschar necrotic skin tissues resulting from burns, corrosive chemicals, or gangrenous wounds.

extensor digitorum muscles that help move fingers or toes. In the lower limbs, the extensor digitorum longus and brevis refer to the long and short extensors of the toes. The belly of the extensor digitorum longus is located in the anterior compartment of the leg and divides into tendons that are distributed to the toes. In the upper limbs, the extensor digitorum communis refers to the common extensor of the digits in the hand located in the posterior compartment of the forearm and also dividing into tendons that attach in the dorsal aspect of the fingers via the extensor hood mechanism.

extensor hallucis the term "hallux" refers to the great toe. Therefore, this muscle is the extensor of the great toe.

extensor retinaculum a band of connective tissue that provides support to the dorsal surface of the wrist and forms a tunnel for the passage of the tendons of the extensor muscles of the wrist and hand.

extensors of the wrist and fingers a group of muscles located in the posterior compartment of the forearm, which attach dorsally and distally to the carpals, metacarpals, and phalanges of the fingers. They are responsible for extending the wrist and the fingers of the hand.

external oblique one of the abdominal muscles located anterolaterally in the abdominal wall and responsible for flexing and rotating the trunk.

extrafusal one of the types of muscle fibers; makes up the bulk of the muscle belly.

exudate the secretions produced as a result of infection or inflammation. In the case of pneumonia, the lungs produce exudate, which settles in the airway and alveoli causing congestion.

facet a flat, hard surface. When the flat, hard surface involves a joint, it is often referred to as an articular facet.

fascia the membranous tissue that covers the muscle and defines the muscle compartments.

flexors of the wrist and finger a group of muscles located in the anterior compartment of the hand, which attach ventrally and distally to the carpals, metacarpals, and phalanges of the fingers. They are responsible for flexing the wrist and fingers.

flexor retinaculum a band of connective tissue that binds the anterior aspect of the wrist from one side to the other. It is also referred as the carpal tunnel because the tendons of the flexors of the fingers and the median nerve course under this structure.

gastrocnemius the muscle that shapes the calf of the leg. It contributes to the formation of the Achilles tendon located distally and posteriorly in the ankle and foot region. It acts primarily as a plantar flexor, but because it originates from above the knee joint, it also helps as a knee flexor.

glenohumeral a connection between the glenoid cavity of the scapula and the humerus, or main bone, of the arm.

goblet cells cells that produce secretions to maintain moisture in the airway.

gluteal referring to the buttock area.

gluteus maximus the muscle that extends the hip and shapes the buttock.

gluteus medius this muscle, along with its partner the gluteus minimus, is located laterally in the hip joint to act as abductor of the hip and also serves to provide support to the hip joint in the standing position.

Golgi tendon organ (GTO) structural portion of a sensory nerve ending, located in tendons, that is responsive to both tension and excessive stretching of muscle tissues. The Golgi tendon organ responds to a quick stretch stimulus by inhibiting the opposite muscle and allowing the primary muscle to act. The Golgi tendon organ is located in the tendinous substance of the muscle. While the muscle spindle facilitates contraction of the agonist, the GTO inhibits activity of the antagonist. If a quick stretch is applied to the biceps brachii muscle in the arm, the muscle spindle is stimulated and the biceps can produce a stronger concentric contraction. Simultaneously, the GTO is activated inhibiting any activity in the antagonist, the triceps muscle. In the case of a muscle spasm, the application of techniques to inhibit hyperactivity of the muscle spindle will simultaneously activate function of the GTO and, consequently, affect contraction in the antagonist.

goniometer an instrument used to measure the degree of movement (angle) of a joint.

gracilis this band-like muscle is one of several muscles that form the adductor group of hip muscles. It is the most superficial of the adductors of the hip.

hematoma a localized collection of blood within an organ or tissue caused by rupture of the blood vessels. Most often the therapist sees a hematoma as a purplish bruise.

hemiparesis weakness on one half or one side of the body.

hemiplegia a condition caused by a cerebrovascular accident involving thrombosis, embolism, or a ruptured aneurysm of one of the arteries that form the Circle of Willis. The result is contralateral paralysis because of the decussation of pathways in the brainstem.

herniation bulging of a structure, as in an intervertebral disc, outside of its normal anatomical location. The varying degrees of bulging can cause compression of the surrounding structures such as nerve roots.

histopathology the study of disease or deterioration of the tissues. It can apply to the integument as well as muscle, connective, myofascial, visceral, or nerve tissues.

humeroulnar joint one of two components of the elbow joint. It is the joint between the olecranon process of the ulna in the forearm, the olecranon fossa of the humerus in the arm, the trocheal of the humerus distally in the arm, and the trochlear notch of the ulna proximally in the forearm.

hypercarbia excessive retention of carbon dioxide in the lungs.

hyperextension excessive extension of a joint allowed under normal circumstances in certain joints of the body, such as the hip and shoulder joints. In certain condyloid or hinge joints, hyperextension is not considered normal and suggests pathology.

hyperreflexia excessive responses to the deep tendon reflexes indicating a clinical problem.

hyperresonance excessive resonance heard when the intercostal spaces of the chest are tapped with a finger. The test is called mediate percussion and is performed to detect a solid, liquid, or gas medium interposed in the chest cavity.

hypertonia excessive tone present in the muscle as a result of trauma or disease of the upper motor neurons. Also referred to as hypertonicity or spasticity.

hypotonia lack of tone in the muscle as a result of trauma or disease of the upper motor neurons. Also called hypotonicity or flaccidity.

iliofemoral ligament the ligament located anteriorly and attaching to the ilium. It is one of the components of the innominate bone of the pelvis and the femur. It is also called the Y ligament of Bigelow because it is shaped like the letter "Y." This ligament is one of the strongest in the body and restricts the extension of the hip.

iliolumbar the ligament or fascia located in the lumbar region and attaching to the iliac crest and the fourth and fifth lumbar vertebrae.

iliopsoas a muscle responsible for flexing the hip joint, which is formed by two components or muscles, the iliacus and the psoas major.

iliotibial band also called the iliotibial tract, a band of connective tissue located along the lateral surface of the thigh.

inflammation one of the body's protective responses to limit tissue damage due to trauma or infectious agents. The body seeks to localize and isolate the damage by dilating arterioles, capillaries, and venules to increase blood flow and to ooze plasma proteins into the localized area. There are three stages of inflammation: acute, subacute, and chronic.

infraspinatus one of the rotator cuff muscles responsible for externally rotating the shoulder joint. The name is derived from its location or origin at the infraspinous fossa of the scapula.

inspiratory the inhalation phase of respiration or breathing.

inspirometer an instrument used to measure the force and volume of inspiration or to train the patient to achieve optimal ventilation during the inspiratory phase.

intercostal located between the ribs.

internal oblique one of the abdominal muscles located anterolaterally in the abdominal wall and responsible for flexing and rotating the trunk to the same side.

interspinous located between the spinous processes of the vertebrae.

intervertebral located between the bodies of the vertebrae.

intrafusal the fibers that are located in and around the immediate vicinity of the muscle spindle.

intrinsic muscles of the hand the muscles that originate and insert within the hand. The small muscles of the thenar eminence in the palm region of the thumb, hypothenar eminence in the palm region of the little finger, and the interosseous muscles located between the metacarpals are examples of intrinsic muscles of the hand. These muscles are fully contained within the hand.

ipsilateral pertaining to the same side.

ischial tuberosity a bony landmark that forms part of the ischium, one of three components of the innominate bone of the pelvis. It is the prominence in the gluteal region on which we sit.

ischiofemoral ligament a ligament that attaches to the ischial tuberosity and the femur.

levator scapulae one of the scapular muscles that attaches to the superior angle of the scapula; named for its function as an elevator of the scapula.

ligamentous referring to the properties of ligaments.

ligamentum flava the ligaments that connect the laminae of the vertebrae along the spine.

ligamentum nuchae a triangular shaped ligament in the extensor surface of the neck that extends from the occipital region at the base of the skull to the spinous process of the seventh cervical vertebra.

linea alba a fibrous band formed as the result of the fusion of the aponeurosis or flat tendon presented by the abdominal muscles where they meet at the center of the abdomen.

lordosis the curve of the lumbar spine.

lubb-dubb the first and second sounds of the heart denoting opening and closing of the heart valves. Clinically, these sounds are referred to as S1 and S2.

lumbodorsal fascia the thick tissue covering the muscles of the lower back.

lumbosacral that which attaches to or covers the region of the lumbar vertebrae and the sacrum.

malalignment defective posture suggesting abnormal alignment of bony segments.

malleoli round, bony prominences, usually referring to the two bony prominences on each side of the ankle joint formed by the tibia and fibula. Each prominence is called a malleolus.

medullary referring to the medulla, the part of the brain at the top of the spinal cord.

MFR abbreviation for myofascial release.

midstance the phase of gait in which the plantar surface of the foot is in total contact with the surface.

midsternum located at the middle of the body of the sternum.

mitral valve the valve that connects the left atrium with the left ventricle of the heart allowing the blood to pass from one chamber to the other.

mobilization the act of manually moving the surfaces of a joint with the objective of improving flexibility and mobility and/or decreasing articular pain.

monoplegia paralysis of one of the four extremities.

multiarticular movements movement in more than one joint or multiple joints at the same time.

multifidus small muscles that form part of the deep layer of muscles of the back, which act as contralateral rotators of the spine.

myocardium relating to the heart muscle. It describes the middle layer of the heart covered by the pericardium on the outside and the endocardium or inner lining on the inside.

nociceptor a pain receptor that relays the message of pain from the skin, soft and connective tissues, or walls of the viscera.

occiput the base of the occipital bone located at the base of the skull.

OOB abbreviation for out of bed; describes a prescribed level of allowed activity.

orthostatic pertains to the upright (or standing) posture or position of the body.

osteokinematics the study of joint movements.

oximeter an instrument that measures the levels or saturation of oxygen in the blood.

patella　commonly known as the knee cap, this is a sesamoid bone contained in the substance of the patellar tendon.

patellar tendon　the tendon of the quadriceps femoris muscle or main extensor of the knee joint.

pathophysiology　describing the loss of function separately from a description of the structural deficits caused by disease or impairment.

pectineus　one of the muscles that form the adductor group of the hip located in the groin area. This is the smallest and most proximal of the hip adductors.

pectoralis major　the primary muscle that covers and shapes the contour of the chest. It is a horizontal adductor of the shoulder originating on the clavicle and sternum and inserting on the humerus.

peripheral chemoreceptor　located in the aorta and common carotid arteries, these are sensors for levels of oxygen in the blood or plasma.

peroneus brevis　a muscle located in the lateral compartment of the leg responsible for eversion or outward movement of the foot.

peroneus longus　covering the peroneus brevis muscle, this is the longest of the two evertors located in the lateral compartment of the leg and causing outward movement of the foot.

pétrissage　a type of massage characterized by kneading of the soft tissue.

piriformis　the largest, strongest, and first of six external rotators of the hip joint originating in the sacrum and inserting laterally in the greater trochanter of the femur. It is located deep in the gluteal region. The sciatic nerve courses under this muscle.

plantaris　one of three muscles located in the superficial layer of the calf. The tendon of this small muscle joins the gastrocnemius and soleus muscles to form the Achilles tendon. This muscle may be absent in 25% of the population.

pneumotaxic center　the respiratory pacemaker; located in the reticular formation of the medulla and the pons. This is one of two respiratory sub-centers responsible for setting the pace between the inspiratory and expiratory phases.

pneumothorax　a pathologic condition characterized by air trapped in the chest cavity. It is caused by rupture of the lung tissue or an opening in the chest such as a stab wound and leads to collapse or atelectasis of the lobe or segment affected.

PNF　an abbreviation that stands for proprioceptive neuromuscular facilitation. It describes a sequence of movements of the upper and lower extremity performed passively or actively following a linear or diagonal pattern and involving all the joints in these extremities.

popliteal　referring to the region or depression in the back of the knee joint.

posterior　located in the back.

postero-anterior　from the back to the front.

post-WaTa　after applying Clinical Wassertanzen maneuvers. See *Wassertanzen*.

prehension　to grasp or grip using the hands.

pre-WaTa　before applying Clinical Wassertanzen maneuvers. See *Wassertanzen*.

pronation a position indicating that the individual is face down or when the palm of the hand moves in and down from the neutral position of thumbs-up so that the palm is facing downward. Pronators are muscles that produce this movement.

pubofemoral ligament a ligament that attaches proximally to the pubic bone, one of three components of the innominate bone of the pelvis, and distally to the femur.

pulmonary bulla air bubble or blister like vesicle formed on the surface of the lungs. If a bulla bursts, air can escape into the chest cavity creating a condition known as pneumothorax. There are other types of bullae; most are distinguished by being filled with fluid and not air, as in the pulmonary bullae.

pulmonic also called pulmonary; used to describe structures associated with the lungs.

radicular denotes association with a spinal nerve root.

radiculopathy a compression or impingement of the spinal nerve root usually resulting in neck or shoulder pain.

radiocarpal joint the joint between the distal radius and two of the carpal bones of the wrist, the lunate and the scaphoid. It forms part of the wrist joint.

Raimeste's technique first described by Brunnstrom in *Movement Therapy in Hemiplegia*. It is a reflex reaction exhibited by patients who have had a stroke. When manual resistance is applied to the unaffected side and the patient is asked to push the segment of the body against resistance, the affected side experiences movement as well to a greater or lesser extent depending on the severity of the cerebrovascular insult.

rale an ambiguous term that generally means a crackling sound in the lungs indicating the presence of secretions in the airway. It is usually considered appropriate to indicate the type of rale heard. Rales are often classified as coarse, medium, and fine, and can be heard at a specific time in the inspiratory phase.

rectus abdominis the most medial and central of the abdominal muscles located in a sheath formed by the aponeurosis of the flat tendon of the oblique muscles.

rectus femoris one of four muscles that collectively form the quadriceps femoris muscle and act primarily as an extensor of the knee. The rectus femoris muscle is the only one of the four that crosses the anterior axis of the hip joint and therefore assists with flexion of the hip as well. The rectus femoris muscle is located centrally on the thigh and, along with the other three components, form the patellar tendon engulfing the patella and finally inserting on the tibial tuberosity.

rhomboid major and minor two scapular muscles that are located medially in the scapula. They attach to the vertebral border of the scapula and the vertebrae and act as adductors of the scapula. Because of the angle of their fibers, at the same time they move the inferior angle of the scapula downwards.

Romberg's test a test used to examine static balance, especially in clients with ataxia. In the first part of the test the client stands with both upper shoulders abducted and eyes closed. Degree of sway is measured. In the second part of the test the client is asked to place the heel of one foot in front of the toes on the other foot. Difference in degree of sway is noted. If the patient demonstrates increased clumsiness, this is a positive sign for peripheral ataxia. If there is no change in the amount of ataxia demonstrated by the client who has ataxia, this indicates that the origin of the ataxia is cerebellar. Some practitioners use only the first part of the test.

sacrospinous ligament a ligament attaching to the spine of the ischium and the sacrum respectively, closing this area to form the greater and lesser sciatic foramina, and providing support to the sacroiliac joint.

sacrotuberous ligament a ligament attaching to the ischial tuberosity and the sacrum respectively, providing support to the sacroiliac joint.

sagittal one of the cardinal planes; divides the body into right and left halves.

sartorius a band-like muscle that crosses the anterior surface of the thigh diagonally. It crosses two joints (the hip and knee) and has multiple actions on both allowing the thigh and leg to flex.

scalenes a group of three muscles in the anterior aspect of the neck responsible for assisting in flexion of the neck but additionally functioning as accessory muscles to respiration because of their insertion on the upper thorax.

scapulohumeral related by connection or direction to the scapula and humerus bones respectively.

scapulothoracic the joint between the scapula resting on the posterior thoracic wall; a relationship between the scapula and thorax.

semilunar valves one of two heart valves that connect the ventricles with the aorta and pulmonary arterial vessels. Their opening ejects blood into systemic and pulmonary circulation.

semimembranosus one of three muscles collectively known as the hamstrings, which acts as the primary flexor of the knee. Because their origin crosses the posterior axis of the hip joint, the hamstrings also act as extensors of the hip joint if their action in the knee joint is isolated.

semispinalis capitis muscle one of the muscles of the spine and back acting as an extensor, this muscle extends to attach in the occipital area.

semitendinosus one of three muscles collectively known as the hamstrings, which act as the primary flexor of the knee. This muscle is adjacent to the semimembranosus and is the most superficial and medial. Because their origin crosses the posterior axis of the hip joint, the hamstrings also act as extensors of the hip joint if their action in the knee joint is isolated.

serratus anterior one of the scapular muscles, which originates on the lateral aspect of the ribs and inserts in the inferior angle of the scapula, therefore acting on upward rotation and abduction of the scapula. It is also considered one of the accessory muscles of respiration as it can pull the ribs outward during the inspiratory phase acting on its origin.

serratus posterior superior and inferior two muscles located in the back under the layer of scapular muscles, which act as accessory muscles of respiration. The serratus posterior superior elevates the ribs during inhalation while the serratus posterior inferior depresses the ribs during exhalation.

SLR an abbreviation that stands for straight leg raise. This is a test for sciatic nerve involvement where the patient is asked to raise the leg with the knee extended and report the onset and intensity of pain or absence of pain.

soft tissue a term that denotes muscle tissue or muscle fibers to differentiate it from myofascial and connective tissue.

soleus one of the calf muscles located directly under the gastrocnemius muscle. It joins the gastrocnemius and plantaris to form the Achilles tendon. Unlike the gastrocnemius, it does not cross the knee joint posteriorly and therefore, only acts as plantar flexor of the ankle.

spasm acute tightening in a group of muscles or muscle fibers. A spasm happens locally and as such can be resolved in a much easier way than spasticity can. For instance, abrupt flexion of the neck during sleep stretches and stimulates the muscle spindle (type II) and causes an abrupt and stronger contraction of a group of fibers in the one or more of the neck extensors (agonists); this creates the muscle "knot" known as the spasm. Concurrently, the alphas (GTO) inhibit the neck flexors (antagonists) allowing the spasm to take place. You wake up with pain and spasms limiting the movement in your neck. Someone gives you a deep tissue massage using an analgesic balm after which you decide to take a warm shower allowing the stream of pulsating water to hydromassage your neck extensors and the spasm goes away. These actions inhibited the tensile sarcomeres in the spasmodic muscle, which resolved the spasm. Contrast with *spasticity*.

spasticity tightening of muscles caused by an impairment of function originating in the central nervous system, usually chronic; not the same as a spasm.

For example, in a CVA, the cerebral insult damages the centers that control muscle tone in such a way that there is a constant state of tension of the myofibril (spasticity), sometimes turning into contractures and deformities. In this case the patient has no control over the degree of spasticity and cannot resolve the problem because of paralysis or weakness. While there are ways to treat spasticity, it is not possible to avoid recurrent episodes unless there is complete healing of the injured CNS centers that control muscle tone. Synonymous with hypertonia or hypertonicity. Contrast with *spasm*.

spinalis the most medial of the components of the erector spinae muscle. It is subdivided according to the regions of the spine it covers along its course into capitis, cervicis, and thoracis.

splenius capitis one of the extensor and ipsilateral rotator muscles of the neck that inserts in the occipital region.

status asthmaticus an acute, severe state of asthma where the patient experiences severe spasms and constriction of the airway.

STR an abbreviation that stands for soft tissue release.

sternoclavicular ligaments ligaments that bind the medial end of the clavicle with the jugular notch of the sternum on each side providing support to this area.

sternocleidomastoid muscle named for its origin on the mastoid process and insertion on the clavicle and sternum, this muscle acts primarily as a contralateral rotator and flexor of the neck but is also considered an accessory muscle of respiration.

subscapularis one of the rotator cuff muscles, which acts as a strong internal rotator of the shoulder. It is named for its origin in the subscapular fossa of the scapula.

subtalar joint the joint between two of the tarsal bones, the inferior surface of the talus or ankle bone and the superior surface of the calcaneus or heel bone. This joint allows side to side motion of the foot. See also *ankle joint*.

sulcus the anatomical description of a long, narrow groove as a landmark in a bone or the brain. Also used to describe a groove in a tooth.

supinator a muscle located superiorly in the forearm, which is responsible for the act of supinating the forearm. Supination is the movement of the hand up and out from the neutral thumbs up position.

supraspinatus one of the rotator cuff muscle responsible for abducting the shoulder joint. Coursing under the coracoacromial ligament, this muscle attaches to the greater tubercle of the humerus.

talocrural joint the joint between the talus, most superior of the tarsal bones, and the crus, or leg, formed by the tibia and fibula. This joint allows dorsiflexion and plantar flexion of the ankle.

tectorial membrane the membrane that marks the attachment of one of the spinal ligaments to the skull at the foramen magnum. It is the terminal end of the posterior longitudinal ligament.

tensor fascia latae a small muscle located in the anterior aspect of the hip inserting on the iliotibial band. This muscle helps rotate the hip medially.

teres major it is considered to be the partner in action of the latissimus dorsi muscle. This is one of the scapular muscles located directly above its partner; acts as an internal rotator of the shoulder.

teres minor considered the partner to the infraspinatus muscle and one of the rotator cuff muscles. This is one of the scapular muscles; located directly below its partner; it acts as external rotator of the shoulder.

thermotherapy treatment using heat. The term "thermo" means "heat" while the term "therapy" means "treatment."

thorac(o)- the thorax or chest.

thoracolumbar pertains to that which is related by connection or direction to the thoracic or chest and lumbar or low back regions.

tibialis anterior a muscle located in the anterior compartment of the leg, which acts primarily as dorsiflexor of the ankle joint.

tibiofemoral joint the joint between the two depressions presented superiorly by the tibia known as the tibial plateau and the two condyles of the femur.

tibiotalar joint the joint between the inferior articular surface of the tibia and the trochlea of the talus, the most superior of the tarsals.

tracheobronchial the trachea, mainstem bronchi, lobar bronchi, and segmental bronchi, essentially denoting the bronchial tree.

transmural through the wall of an organ. The prefix "trans" means "across" while "mural" means "wall."

trapezius one of the scapular muscles. This muscle is so named because of its shape. It covers a considerable range of the upper scapular and neck regions. It is divided into three portions each of which has an individual action. The upper trapezius is an elevator of the shoulder; the middle trapezius retracts the scapula; the lower trapezius depresses the scapula.

Trendelenburg gait a gait pattern typically exhibited by patients with unilaterally weak hip abductors. When the gluteus medius and minimus are weak, the patient tends to experience a lateral trunk lean on the contralateral side of the weakness.

triceps brachii the muscle that acts as the main extensor of the elbow joint, inserting on the olecranon process and originating high on the shoulder. It is called triceps because it has three heads of origin, one of which crosses the shoulder joint posteriorly and assists with shoulder extension.

triceps surae a term used to designate the two heads of the gastrocnemius and one origin of the soleus as one muscular unit.

ulnar associated by connection, direction, or location to the medial (ulna) aspect of the arm.

vasodilation opening up or expansion of an arterial or venous vessel. Vasodilation can be induced by heat or through medications.

vastus lateralis one of four muscles that collectively form the quadriceps femoris muscle and act primarily as an extensor of the knee. The vastus lateralis muscle is located laterally on the thigh and, along with the other three components, forms the patellar tendon engulfing the patella and finally inserting on the tibial tuberosity.

vastus medialis one of four muscles that collectively form the quadriceps femoris muscle and act primarily as an extensor of the knee. The vastus medialis, also known as vastus medialis oblique because of the orientation of muscle fibers, is located medially on the thigh and, along with the other three components, forms the patellar tendon engulfing the patella and finally inserting on the tibial tuberosity.

ventilatory capacity the capacity of the lungs to intake a volume of air with an adequate amount of oxygen to properly ventilate the dependent areas of the lungs, particularly at the bases of the lungs.

walker an assistive ambulatory device used when partial weight bearing unilaterally or bilaterally is indicated. It consists of a fence-like device with four legs that remain in contact with the surface and two hand bars.

Wassertanzen a set of maneuvers used in aquatic therapy. Literally (from the German) "Water Dancing."

WaTa an abbreviation that stands for Wassertanzen.

Watsu® Created by Harold Dull at Harbin Hot Springs, California; an aquatic therapy intervention that integrates applied shiatsu techniques into the aquatic environment in a series of movement or positional sequences or flows.

xyphoid a sharp pointed process that marks the inferior end of the sternum. It is cartilaginous through the early adult stages of life ossifying at age 40 or older.

zygapophyseal joints known as the posterior intervertebral joints, these are the joints between the superior and inferior articular facets of the vertebrae in the spine. The union of these facets forms the intervertebral foramen through which the spinal nerve root exits.

REFERENCES

Amsterdam, E. A., Willmore, J. H., & DeMaria, A. N. (1977). *Exercise in cardiovascular health and disease.* New York: Yorke Medical Books, Dunn-Donnelley Publishing Corporation.

Bates, A. & Hanson, N. (1996). *Aquatic exercise therapy.* Philadelphia, PA: W. Saunders Company.

Bourdillon, J. F. & Day, E. A. (1987). *Spinal manipulation* (4th ed.). Appleton & Lange.

Boyle, A. M. (1981). The Bad Ragaz ring method. *Physiotherapy*, Vol. 67, No. 9.

Brannon, F. J., Foley, M. W., Starr, J. A., & Saul, L. M. (1998). *Cardiopulmonary rehabilitation: Basic theory and application* (3rd ed.). Philadelphia, PA: F. A. Davis Company.

Bullock, B. L. (1996). *Pathophysiology: Adaptations and alterations in functions* (4th ed.). New York: B. Lippincott Company.

Cantu, R. I. & Grodin, A. J. (1992). *Myofascial manipulation: Theory and clinical application.* Gaithersburg, MD: Aspen Publications.

Chusid, J. G. (1973). *Correlative neuroanatomy and functional neurology* (15th ed.). Lange Medical Publications.

Cunningham, J. (1997). Halliwick method. In R. G. Ruoti, D. M. Morris, & A. J. Cole. (Eds.). *Aquatic rehabilitation.* Philadelphia, PA: B. Lippincott Company.

Dull, H. (1997). *Watsu: Freeing the body in water* (2nd ed.). Middletown, CA: Harbin Springs Publishing.

Erickson, B. (1991). *Heart sounds and murmurs: A practical guide* (2nd ed.). Philadelphia, PA: Mosby Yearbook Medical Publishers.

Frownfelter, D., & Dean, E. (1996). *Principles and practice of cardiopulmonary therapy* (3rd ed.). Philadelphia, PA: Mosby Yearbook Medical Publishers.

Garret, G. (1997). Bad Ragaz ring method. In R. G. Ruoti, D. M. Morris, & A. J. Cole. (Eds.). *Aquatic rehabilitation.* Philadelphia, PA: B. Lippincott Company.

Hertling, D. & Kessler, R. M. (1990). *Management of common musculoskeletal disorders: Therapy principles and methods* (2nd ed.). Philadelphia, PA: B. Lippincott Company.

Kaplan, P. E. & Tanner, E. D. (1989). *Musculoskeletal pain and disability.* Appleton & Lange.

Lundy-Ekman, L. (1998). *Neuroscience: Fundamentals for rehabilitation*. Philadelphia, PA: W. B. Saunders Company.

Michlovitz, S. (1990). *Thermal agents in rehabilitation*. Philadelphia, PA: F. A. Davis Company.

Norkin, C. C. & Levangie, P. K. (1992). *Joint structure and function: A comprehensive analysis* (2nd ed.). Philadelphia, PA: F. A. Davis Company.

Pollock, M. L., Wilmore, J. H., & Fox III, S. M. (1984). *Exercise in health and disease: Evaluation and prescription for prevention and rehabilitation*. Philadelphia, PA: W. B. Saunders Company.

Ruoti, R. G., Morris, D. M., & Cole, A. J. (1997). *Aquatic rehabilitation*. Philadelphia, PA: B. Lippincott Company.

Sherman, C. (1992). Managing fibromyalgia with exercise. *The Physician and Sports Medicine*, Vol. 20, No. 10, pp. 166-172.

Smith, L. K., Weiss, E. L., & Lehmkuhl, L. D. (1996). *Brunnstrom's clinical kinesiology* (5th ed.). Philadelphia, PA: F. A. Davis Company.

INDEX

ABOUT THE AUTHOR

Dr. Luis G. Vargas received his Master of Education Degree in Educational Administration from Cambridge College. He received his doctorate degree from the Higher Education Administration at The Union Institute's Graduate School in Cincinnati, Ohio, in 1990.

He has chaired several academic programs in physical therapy including his current position as Associate Professor at Hamilton University. His areas of expertise as an academic educator include human gross anatomy, pathophysiology, biomechanics, diagnostic assessment, pulmonary physical therapy, cardiac rehabilitation, infectious disease, oncology, physical agents, and aquatic rehabilitation.

He is a certified Watsu Practitioner and has completed training in levels I and II Wassertanzen. His critical analysis and study of the effectiveness of these approaches to treatment in various orthopedic, neurological, and cardiopulmonary conditions led to the development of his Diagnostic Aquatics Systems Integration Theory, which established a clinico-pathologic relevance between the interventions used in aquatic therapy and their physiological effects. The foundations established by Dr. Vargas gave rise to his aquatic movement science theory, which served as the basis from which he designed and developed other interventions and protocols such as his Cardiaquatics Protocol for the partially rehabilitated cardiac or risk-factor patient, and his Clinical Wassertanzen Protocol.

Dr. Vargas has also analyzed the arthrokinematic and physiological effects of Watsu and Ai Chi on soft tissue structures. Based on his analysis, he formulated the theories and three phases of breathing control that served as the foundation for his three-phase Clinical Wassertanzen Protocol based on his synthesis of the original European aquatic bodywork program.

Dr. Vargas introduced aquatic rehabilitation as a clinical specialty to the Commonwealth of Puerto Rico where he continues to conduct training workshops for the Puerto Rican physical therapy community. He was a presenter at the 2002 and 2003 International Congress of Physical Therapy in Costa Rica where he continues to collaborate as Consultant to the Universidad Santa Paula, School of Physical Therapy.

He is the recipient of the 2000 Dolphin Award by the Aquatic Therapy and Rehabilitation Institute at that year's annual symposium held in Orlando, Florida. He continues to serve as an active member of the faculty for the Aquatic Therapy and Rehabilitation Institute conducting professional seminars, specialty institute workshops, and presentations at symposia. He also serves on various committees for this agency and has intensified his efforts regarding the credentialing process for aquatic rehabilitation practitioners.

Dr. Luis G. Vargas is the founder, President, and CEO of *Aquatica, Inc.*, a company committed to the further development and establishment of Aquatic Rehabilitation as a clinical specialty through his training programs and specialty workshops for various healthcare disciplines, through his continued professional consultation services as expert to clinics throughout the United States and the world, through his ongoing research, and through his design and implementation of protocols and interventions and the manufacturing of products for the industry.